DIABETES
RESCUE
DIET

DIABETES
RESCUE
DIET

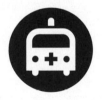

Conquer Diabetes Naturally
While Eating and Drinking
What You Love—
Even Chocolate and Wine!

MARK BRICKLIN
former editor-in-chief of **Prevention**®

RODALE.

Book design by Carol Angstadt

Library of Congress Cataloging-in-Publication Data
Bricklin, Mark.
    Diabetes rescue diet : Conquer diabetes naturally while eating and drinking what you
love—even chocolate and wine! / Mark Bricklin.
        p.   cm.
    ISBN 978-1-60961-768-4 (direct hardcover)
    1. Diabetes—Diet therapy—Popular works.   2. Diabetes—Nutritional aspects—Popular
works.   3. Self-care, Health—Popular works.   I. Title.
    RC662.B74   2012
    616.4'620654—dc23   2011047526

2   4   6   8   10   9   7   5   3   1   hardcover

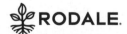

RODALE.

We inspire and enable people to improve their lives and the world around them.
For more of our products visit rodalestore.com or call 800-848-4735.

To my wife, Lynn, whose love and encouragement
made this book possible

Acknowledgments

I'd like to express my gratitude to my editorial associate,
Julia VanTine, for her invaluable contributions.

Contents

Introduction

What if it were so easy to prevent diabetes that you didn't need a special diet at all? What if the food you eat every day could reduce your risk of this epidemic disease by more than 80 percent?

That was the conclusion of a large study that found people who just naturally ate in a certain pattern were largely "immune" to diabetes, compared with others of the same age and background who ate in a different way. The reduction in risk was more dramatic than that seen with any doctor-prescribed program, including prescription drugs (even when combined with exercise).

The protective eating pattern these researchers studied is known as the Mediterranean diet, and when people are instructed to follow its principles, the results are stunning: lower incidence of diabetes, fewer complications, less need for medications, and much more.

This diet—which really isn't a diet at all but a general pattern of food selection—originally came to the attention of medical researchers 50 or 60 years ago, when they found that people who ate this way had a remarkably lower rate of heart disease than people who followed more Western or "modern" diets.

Only recently have researchers discovered that this same traditional "menu" also protects against diabetes. And since the number one health threat to people with diabetes is heart disease, we're looking at double protection from one diet!

The Diabetes Rescue Diet is based on the traditional Mediterranean diet, so you know you're getting massive health protection. But this plan goes beyond the basics: I've made a few tweaks—I'm talking small, easy-to-follow changes—that supercharge the diet to provide even more protection. As you'll read in Part 1, a leading nutrition and health expert says that the Diabetes Rescue Diet could reduce the risk of diabetes by as much as 90 percent!

The Rescuers Work Together

As I researched this book, I found that scientists all over the world are trying to dissect the Mediterranean diet and discover what makes it tick. Their goal is to find one or more particular compounds that can be put into pill form to be sold like statin drugs.

But it looks to me like they're missing the point: These benefits don't come from one magic ingredient but the whole dietary pattern. And some experts believe the foods featured in the Mediterranean diet don't promote health all by themselves but, rather, interact with one another in a way that makes the sum much greater than the parts.

A Plan You'll Love to Live With

I've been a health journalist for more than 40 years. And to me, the most remarkable thing about the Diabetes Rescue Diet is not how powerful its ingredients are but how easy it is to follow. That's crucial, because to be perfectly honest, most—maybe all—ideas about how to prevent diabetes fail in real life because the majority of people simply cannot follow them.

For example, the number one standard piece of advice on avoiding diabetes is to lose weight. That's a good idea, but as you'll see later, the success rate of weight-loss diets over the long term is pathetically low. For people who already have diabetes, the real-life possibility of losing weight is even lower.

Studies prove that you don't have to drop pounds to reduce your risk of diabetes. And while exercise greatly benefits your body and mind (I highly recommend it!), it isn't essential to reducing your risk of diabetes.

Then there are the foods you can and can't eat. One popular diet today, urged for weight loss and diabetes protection, is the low-carbohydrate diet. It should really be called the *no*-carbohydrate diet, because with the classic prescription, you can't eat bread (not even whole grain), oatmeal, cereal, rolls, pasta, rice, potatoes, polenta, or corn on the cob (not to mention *pizza*!). Most people can't stick with such a superstrict regimen. Could you?

Another diet promoted for defending against diabetes requires zero consumption of meat, fish, poultry, eggs, cheese, yogurt, or any other dairy products. Plus, you can't put vegetable oil on that huge salad. Ready to dig in? Me neither.

Not all diets are so extreme. The widely prescribed "prudent" or low-fat diets allow more leeway, but—as you'll read later—in head-to-head real-life trials against Mediterranean-style diets, they consistently lose when it comes to measured health benefits.

Why This Will Work for You

The Diabetes Rescue Diet will be easy for you to follow for several reasons.

★ *It's truly delicious!* Not pretend delicious, the way restricted diets describe themselves, but gourmet delicious from soup to nuts, from wine to coffee. How does Orange-Beef Stir-Fry (page 216) sound? Or Raspberry-Almond Cheesecake (page 240)? They're both on our list of recipes—and you can easily make hundreds of your own favorites as part of the plan.

★ *It's positive, not negative!* All the other diets I've looked at demand serious cuts or absolute omission of the foods and ingredients that people like most—no fat, no salt, no carbs, no starch. Overwhelmingly, the research I've read on the proven benefits of the Mediterranean diet measures adherence by how many good foods you eat, not how many "bad" foods you eat.

★ *It's easy to understand!* When I was editor of *Prevention* and founding editor of *Men's Health*, the world's two most widely read health magazines, I insisted that the staff not write anything that the average person couldn't understand—even if quoting the advice of a health expert. A perfect example is nutritionists' oft-repeated advice that one should not get more than 30 percent of their daily calories from fat. Do you have any idea what percentage of your total calories come from fat? No one does! Yet this "advice" is given over and over again. Another common piece of meaningless advice is to eat 30 grams of fiber a day. Most Americans don't even know what a gram is. (There are 28 of them in 1 ounce—now you know.) In the Diabetes Rescue Diet, there are no magic percentages and no grams to measure. There are just foods to eat, with a target number of servings a day. The foods naturally supply all the vitamins, minerals, fiber, protein, antioxidants, and other nutrients you want for optimum health. You won't need a scale, computer, or laboratory to know if you're on the right track.

★ *No need to lose weight or count calories!* I mentioned above that the Diabetes Rescue Diet works even in the absence of weight loss. That's because it's the food's nutrients—not the calories—that are associated with protecting against diabetes. Common sense says you're better off not eating excessive portions of foods, no matter what they are. But you'll feel satisfied with a belly full of the fruits, vegetables, beans, fish, and other foods that are the backbone of your new eating plan. As you'll read later, the Diabetes Rescue Diet encourages weight control naturally.

★ *No weirdness!* There are no supplements, herbs, powders, or potions involved. No need to eat six times a day. No quick-start period. No cleansing procedures. No cheat days. No baloney. You'll be eating the most natural diet imaginable!

★ *No need for perfection!* Suppose you simply don't like some the foods emphasized in our diet. Not to worry! Later you'll read about a trial conducted in India, where some of the key ingredients of the Mediterranean diet are either not available or are forbidden by local custom. So researchers modified the diet and still achieved spectacular results, compared with a standard low-fat diet.

★ *Long-term results!* This is one of the only diet books that doesn't promise you'll "lose 20 pounds in 20 days," "see results in 10 days," or "change your metabolism [and dress size, appetite, and fingerprints] in 5 days." Why? Because there's no need for such exaggerated claims. The benefits of this diet have been nailed down by a host of real-life studies and trials involving thousands of people all over the world.

And these benefits are all long-term, most lasting years, not weeks or even months. I can't emphasize enough how important that is. Short-term trials are notorious for long-term failure. Once the blitz is over, people relapse into their old ways. With the Diabetes Rescue Diet, there is no blitz—just a very normal, easy eating plan that science and medicine have shown results in remarkable and lasting health protection.

This Diet Works Overtime!

One of the most fascinating discoveries I made in researching this book is that besides protecting against diabetes and its number one complication, heart disease, the Mediterranean diet also protects against a wide range of other problems, many of them serious and all too common.

I was so impressed by this that I devoted Part 3 of this book to Shortcuts and Healthy Bonuses. I hope you read it, because this information has never before been gathered in one place.

Some of these bonuses are not exactly shocking. I mean, if the diet protects against heart disease, you'd suspect it would also protect against high blood pressure, since the two are so closely related. And it does.

But cancer? Rheumatoid arthritis? Gallstone disease? Serious depression? Asthma? Even Alzheimer's disease?

Most people wouldn't suspect a relationship between diet and these health problems, except maybe for cancer. But the benefits of the Mediterranean diet and its key components can be huge. For example, this eating style has been shown to reduce the risk of Alzheimer's disease by more than two-thirds!

How can one simple eating plan, with so few rules, protect against so many illnesses involving not just your sugar metabolism but your nerves, brain, liver, lungs, and more? No one really knows. But it's pretty obvious that there's something about this diet that is profoundly right for health at every level and maybe for every tissue in the body. You get the full reward with the Diabetes Rescue Diet!

Part 1

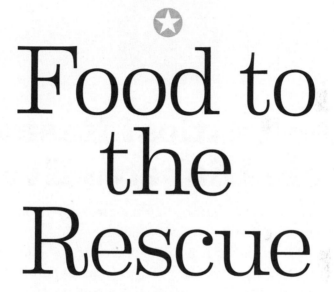

Food to the Rescue

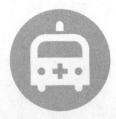

The Tastiest Rescue from Diabetes Ever

Lois Lane had Superman. Timmy had Lassie. And if you have or are at risk of diabetes, I've come to rescue *you*.

If you need to be saved from the specter of diabetes—the more common type 2 variety, which evidence links to being overweight and living an unhealthy lifestyle—you're not alone. In just 30 years, the number of people with diabetes worldwide has more than doubled, exploding from 153 million in 1980 to 347 million in 2008, a team of American and British scientists found. Their research, published in the medical journal the *Lancet*, comes from blood samples taken from almost three million people ages 25 and up from around the world.

More alarming, just being American seems to be a risk factor. The number of Americans who develop diabetes is rising twice as fast as the number of Western Europeans who do, the study found. Nearly 26 million Americans have type 2 diabetes. That's more people than in the states of Pennsylvania and Illinois combined!

Another 79 million have prediabetes, which raises the risk of developing full-blown diabetes. And untold millions don't even know they have blood sugar problems. This is alarming because diabetes can sneak up on you suddenly—and left unchecked, the disease can affect your vision, your longevity, and certainly your quality of life.

Type 2 diabetes is the leading cause of blindness and kidney failure, and adults with diabetes have heart disease death rates two to four times higher than those without diabetes. People with diabetes are two to four times more likely to be felled by a stroke, too.

But it doesn't have to be this way for you. Never fear—the Diabetes Rescue Diet is here!

Many diet and lifestyle plans promise to prevent diabetes and its complications, so why does the diabetes rate keep climbing? And among those who have the disease, why does control of blood sugar seem to be getting worse?

As I see it, the problem is that most diabetes plans are too hard to follow. Typically, they insist that you lose weight, cut out almost all fat, or virtually eliminate bread, pasta, grains, or all but a smidgen of fruit from your diet.

I know I can't follow a diet that forbids meat, eggs, and cheese or that says I can't have milk and fruit on my cereal or olive oil on my salad. Luckily, there's a plan that I not only can follow but *want* to follow—and I'm pretty sure you will, too. It's a delicious and very healthy plan that a large part of the world has followed for centuries.

The "Diabetes Diet" That Isn't

The Diabetes Rescue Diet is based almost entirely on the traditional Mediterranean diet, a pattern of eating followed in certain countries around the Mediterranean Sea, including Italy, Spain, and Greece. In the mid-1990s, researchers at Harvard Medical School began publishing their findings on the Mediterranean way of eating, which showed that it greatly reduced the risk of heart disease.

More recently, researchers have focused on the benefits of the Mediterranean way of eating on diabetes and found this same diet to be a powerful protector. In fact, researchers have found the Mediterranean diet to be such an ideal model for preventing and managing diabetes that I just have to call attention to a few of their conclusions—you'll find quotes from these prestigious studies scattered throughout this chapter.

The Diabetes Rescue Diet remains so close to the Mediterranean diet that it shares all the research-based benefits, but I've added in practices designed to supercharge your protection.

The eating plan is so simple that I can sketch the basics in one paragraph: more fruits, vegetables, salads, whole grains, beans, fish, seafood, and nuts; small to moderate amounts of wine (only if you're comfortable with that); the use of olive oil as the only added fat; moderate to generous amounts of low-fat dairy products; and less meat and junk food.

You don't have to follow these guidelines perfectly—just shifting your diet in the right direction helps. Basically, it's a more-of-this, less-of-that diet. Nothing is absolutely excluded, though you'll very rarely be eating bacon double cheeseburgers with fries and a Coke!

There's no need to count calories, weigh your food, take supplements, eat six times a day, or follow any of those annoying "musts." Nor do you have to buy your food in ethnic markets or even eat stereotypical Mediterranean fare such as hummus, olives, or feta cheese. You can find all the ingredients you'll need at your local grocery store, and you may be surprised by how many of your favorite foods are still on the menu. I'll show you how to enjoy all the proven benefits of this diet while eating in a way that makes you happy.

Delicious and satisfying, recipes from the Diabetes Rescue Diet can even be served to your family and friends or at parties—to rave reviews! You can purchase the makings at any decent supermarket and find foods from the diet on any first-rate restaurant menu.

The Diabetes Rescue Diet can do more than help you avoid diabetes—it can help you launch a more vibrant life. If you've been recently diagnosed, this program may help you reverse the disease. Lived with diabetes for years? This plan can help you take control of your health for good. But let's review the basics: what diabetes is and what science has discovered about it in recent years.

The History of the Mediterranean Diet

When we talk about the Mediterranean diet, we mean the traditional diet of the people who lived around this beautiful, island-dotted sea, particularly the Greeks and Italians.

For centuries, these folks farmed the land, turning the grapes and olives they grew into wine and olive oil. Because the climate is not right for grazing animals, these people didn't eat beef or much dairy. What they did eat were fruits, vegetables, olives and olive oil, nuts, and fish. If they ate meat, milk, or cheese, it typically came from goats.

In the 1940s, an American nutritionist named Ancel Keys noticed that men who lived in the mountains of Crete and ate a traditional Cretan diet of grains, vegetables, beans, fruits, and olive oil had low rates of heart disease and cancer, and lived to a very old age. Intrigued, he wanted to find out why.

The now-famous (and still ongoing) Seven Countries Study, which began in 1958, initially involved almost 13,000 middle-aged men and looked at the relationship between diet and disease. Results showed that men who followed a Mediterranean diet had less coronary heart disease. This and later studies indicated that a diet low in saturated fat can reduce cholesterol and the risk of heart disease. (More than half the fat in a Mediterranean diet is the monounsaturated variety, mainly from olive oil.)

Then, in the mid-1990s, the Harvard School of Public Health, the European Office of the World Health Organization, and the nonprofit Oldways organization introduced the traditional Mediterranean diet. Walter Willett, MD, of Harvard, along with his colleagues, developed the Mediterranean diet pyramid, and he has become the modern face of a traditional, delicious, and very healthy way of eating.

One thing to keep in mind: The eating plan described in this book is based on the *traditional* Mediterranean way of eating. Sadly, the diet in this region is becoming more westernized (dare we say McDonaldized?), and the people are paying for it—with rising rates of diabetes. Fortunately, the traditional Mediterranean-style diet still works, and to benefit, all you have to do is enjoy it!

Big Gains in Health—
Even If the Scale Is Stuck

If you have or are at risk of diabetes, most doctors will tell you to take off weight. Of course, that's sound advice if you can do it! But even if you can't, here's the best news: Time and again, all over the world, the Mediterranean diet has been shown to stop diabetes in its tracks—without the need for weight loss or added exercise. Consider the results of these major studies. The Mediterranean diet:

★ **Reduces the risk of prediabetes.** A 2011 analysis of results from 50 different studies involving more than half a million people, reported in the *Journal of the American College of Cardiology,* found that the Mediterranean diet can prevent a prediabetic condition called metabolic syndrome. The results showed that adherence to the diet was associated with smaller waistlines, lower blood pressure, and lower blood sugar and cholesterol levels—leading to a 31 percent reduction in the risk of developing metabolic syndrome and, thus, lower risk of diabetes.

★ **Reduces the development of diabetes itself.** In one major study reported in the *British Medical Journal,* researchers from Spain assessed the eating habits of almost 14,000 university alumni. Using a detailed food-frequency questionnaire that covered more than 130 different foods and scored on a 9-point index, the researchers tracked these alums' eating habits for more than 4 years. They found that those who followed the Mediterranean way of eating most closely—scoring between 7 and 9 on the index—reduced their risk of developing diabetes by an incredible 83 percent!

★ **Reduces the complications of diabetes**—especially heart disease, the number one threat to people with diabetes. In a study conducted in Australia, researchers gauged the eating patterns of more than 40,000 men and women ages 40 to 69, again by assessing food questionnaires. After tracking these folks for 10 years, the researchers found that, compared with those who ate the least amount of Mediterranean-diet foods, those who ate the most lowered their risk of dying from coronary heart disease by a mind-blowing 79 percent!

★ **Helps all older people live longer.** A team of researchers from the Netherlands, Spain, and Rome set out to investigate the effect of the healthy Mediterranean diet and lifestyle on deaths from all causes—including heart disease, cancer, and cardiovascular disease—in more than 2,000 elderly Europeans. When the study began in 1988, the participants were all over age 70, and some were as old as 90. The researchers tracked them for 10 years. The results of the study—published in 2004 in the *Journal of the American Medical Association*—found that those who stuck closest to a Mediterranean diet and lifestyle lowered their risk of death from all causes by more than 50 percent.

Again, although it's smart to lose weight and exercise if you have or are at risk of diabetes, the studies above prove that the Mediterranean way of eating gives you all these benefits without the need to do either. But it does even more. As you'll read in Part 3, going Mediterranean also promotes a marked reduction in a number of diseases besides diabetes, including obesity, high blood pressure, cancer, and Alzheimer's disease.

The Diabetes Rescue Diet:
A "Real World" Solution

The Diabetes Rescue Diet isn't the only program that has proven successful in turning back diabetes. It's just the *best*. The main reason: It's doable. So doable that you can start it today and begin improving your health by bedtime.

Other approaches are much more difficult. Take the Finnish Diabetes Prevention Study, for example. It's one of the best known of the diabetes prevention programs. Hundreds of people with impaired blood sugar control and other conditions that put them at higher risk of developing diabetes were able to reduce their risk by 58 percent over a 4-year intervention period, compared with a similar group that did nothing special. This study is often cited as proof that a few simple lifestyle changes can protect you. But it certainly wasn't the most enjoyable way to reduce diabetes risk.

First, all of the participants were put on calorie-restricted, high-fiber, low-fat diets. Of course, they had a little help. Each person had seven one-on-one sessions with a nutritionist during the first year of the study, and three more every year until the study ended after 4 years. That's nearly 20 sessions.

But wait, it gets better. They also got personal guidance on increasing their physical activity. Did they like to swim? Ski? Walk? Whatever their choice, they were encouraged and coached. On top of that, they were enrolled in supervised, progressive, individualized resistance-training classes—weight lifting with a personal trainer, basically. And no lollygagging: They were urged to do a moderate to high number of repetitions on a circuit of exercises. Plus, they got regular health checkups.

Accentuate the Positive

66 It appears more important to increase the number of healthy foods regularly consumed than to reduce the number of less healthy foods regularly consumed."

That's the conclusion of a study that looked at the diet and health of some 59,000 Swedish women. These women, who ate a wide variety of healthy foods over the years, were found to have an amazing 42 percent lower risk of dying from any and all causes than those who ate few healthy foods.

What were those "healthy foods"? A diverse assortment of fruits, vegetables, whole grain breads, cereals, fish, and low-fat dairy—precisely the foods featured in the Diabetes Rescue Diet.

The interesting thing is that this study found it was much more important to eat more of those healthy foods than to worry about avoiding unhealthy ones, including red meats, refined carbs, and foods high in saturated fat. That's the same approach we emphasize: Accentuate the positive and worry less about eliminating the negative.

Can you even imagine finding a program like this? In the event you did, can you imagine sticking with it for 4 years? With an estimated 79 million Americans having prediabetes, along with the increasing pressures to reduce health care costs, let's be realistic. If it would cost just $1,000 a year for each at-risk person, the price tag for 4 years would be more than $300 billion! It's a wonderful idea, but it ain't gonna happen.

The Diabetes Rescue Diet is a real-world solution, not a fantasy. It is proven to prevent diabetes and its complications, and does not require weight loss (like the Finnish study does), one-on-one sessions with a nutritionist, or progressive (harder and harder) supervised exercise. It doesn't even require a low-fat diet.

Stopping Diabetes in Its Tracks

Type 2 diabetes, the most common kind by far, begins long before you get an official diagnosis from your doctor. It's often preceded by metabolic syndrome, which leads not just to diabetes but to heart disease as well. And this condition is scarily widespread.

One out of every three people in America has metabolic syndrome. Worse, 44 percent of people over age 50 in the United States have this dangerous condition, which pushes their risk of diabetes five times higher. In fact, 85 percent of people with diabetes also have metabolic syndrome.

Metabolic syndrome really gets rolling in middle age: 41 percent of men and 37 percent of women ages 40 to 59 have this condition, as do 52 percent of men and 54 percent of women over age 60. Doctors diagnose it when someone has three or more of the following five conditions:

★ Blood pressure equal to or higher than 130/85

★ Fasting blood glucose equal to or higher than 100 mg/dL

★ A waistline measuring 35 inches or more in women and 40 inches or more in men

★ HDL (high-density lipoprotein, or "good") cholesterol under 40 in men and under 50 in women

★ Triglycerides equal to or higher than 150 mg/dL

The good news, as I already mentioned briefly, is that the Mediterranean diet has been shown to knock out metabolic syndrome, too. Reporting in the *American Journal of Cardiology,* researchers from Greece and Italy reviewed the results of 50 published studies with more than 500,000 participants as part of a meta-analysis—a statistical analysis of the findings of similar studies—on the Mediterranean diet. Among their findings: The Mediterranean style of eating is associated with a lower risk of hikes in blood pressure, blood sugar, and

Diabetes Comes in Two "Flavors"

Chances are, if you're reading this book, you have type 2 diabetes—the most common variety, which is linked to being overweight and having an unhealthy lifestyle. But there's also another kind: type 1 diabetes. While both types cause blood sugar levels to become higher than normal, they do so in different ways.

Type 1 diabetes (formerly known as insulin-dependent, or juvenile, diabetes) occurs when the immune system attacks and destroys the cells of the pancreas that produce the hormone insulin. People with type 1 need insulin to help keep their blood sugar levels within a normal range.

Unlike someone with type 1, a person with type 2 diabetes (which used to be called non-insulin-dependent diabetes) still produces insulin—but the body doesn't respond to it normally. Glucose is less able to enter the cells and do its job of supplying energy. This is called insulin resistance, and it causes blood sugar levels to rise, making the pancreas produce even more insulin. Eventually, the pancreas can wear out from working overtime and may no longer be able to make enough of the hormone to keep blood sugar levels normal.

People with insulin resistance may or may not develop type 2 diabetes; it depends on whether the pancreas can produce enough insulin to keep blood sugar levels normal. Repeatedly high blood sugar levels, however, suggest type 2 diabetes. A normal fasting blood sugar level is less than 100 milligrams per deciliter (mg/dL). A fasting blood sugar level between 100 and 125 mg/dL is considered prediabetes; 126 mg/dL or higher is considered diabetes.

triglycerides, as well as a reduced risk of a drop in good cholesterol—all of which are risk factors for metabolic syndrome.

There's really no surprise here—many studies have confirmed the role of the Mediterranean diet in reducing heart disease. So it makes sense that the diet would also reduce the risks that lead up to heart disease.

The point I'm trying to make is that, yes, you want to guard your health against diabetes. But to do that, you also want to stave off metabolic syndrome—and eating like Zorba the Greek is a simple, smart, and satisfying way to do it.

Diabetes Reduced by 83 Percent!

As I've discussed, the earliest signs of diabetes can be reversed with the Diabetes Rescue Diet. What about diabetes itself?

Let me return to the study by researchers in Spain. Its findings were nothing short of spectacular. The team found that moderate adherence to the Mediterranean diet correlated with a 59 percent lower risk of diabetes—and highest adherence (the top third of participants) with an 83 percent lower risk.

Keep in mind, these people who greatly reduced their risk of diabetes weren't even on any kind of diet. They just ate that way naturally, proving that our diet is eminently doable.

The authors of this study also pointed out something interesting: Participants who stuck most closely to the Mediterranean way of eating were more likely to have important risk factors for diabetes—they tended to be older and had a higher body mass index (a measure of fatness), family history of diabetes, and personal history of high blood pressure. There was also a higher proportion of ex-smokers. Therefore, the authors of the study would have expected to find a higher incidence of diabetes among these participants—but no. Although at higher risk, these Mediterranean diet "diehards" actually had a lower risk of diabetes, suggesting that their eating style might have a substantial potential for prevention.

You don't even need to lose weight or do strenuous exercise to lower your risk of diabetes. Another study called PREDIMED prescribed different diets to people. Researchers put a control group on a low-fat diet and assigned the rest of the participants to one of two Mediterranean diets, supplemented with one of two Mediterranean staples: virgin olive oil (34 ounces of the stuff a week!) or nuts (around an ounce a day). Compared with the control diet, the other two diets cut diabetes risk by 52 percent.

The key point of this study is that *diabetes risk reduction occurred in the absence of significant changes in body weight or physical activity.* This is of crucial importance, because in the real world, as we'll see later, people find it difficult to lose weight or keep it off, and many don't exercise.

Less Medication Needed!

For most people, it's simply easier to pop a pill than to make positive lifestyle changes.

But here's a fact you've never heard before: As people take more drugs—and rely less on diet—their blood sugar control significantly dwindles.

Researchers looked at data from two major studies—called the National Health and Nutrition Examination Surveys—which were conducted in 1988 and again in 2000. They found that during those 12 years, the use of diet as the only therapy for diabetes declined from 27 percent to 20 percent. At the same time, the use of oral antidiabetes drugs increased from 45 to 52 percent. Let me repeat that: Diet therapy went down 7 points; drugs, up 7 points.

Meanwhile, the percentage of people with diabetes whose blood sugar was under control dropped from 44.5 percent to 35.8 percent. That's a drop of 19 percent!

Blood sugar control is the keystone of diabetes treatment, and if you are living with diabetes now, our plan can help right from the get-go. In a study conducted by researchers from Italy and the United Kingdom, more than 200 people with newly diagnosed type 2 diabetes were put on one of two diets. The first was a Mediterranean-style plan, which got half of its daily calories from carbohydrates. The second plan was a typical low-fat diet, with 30 percent of daily calories coming from fat. The researchers followed both groups for 4 years.

At the end of the study, the group assigned to the Mediterranean-style plan had better blood sugar control and were less likely to need oral medications to control blood sugar than those assigned to the low-fat diet. Specifically, less than half of the people in the Mediterranean-style group—44 percent—needed medication, compared with 70 percent in the low-fat group.

But that's not all. Those assigned to the Mediterranean-style diet

Defeating Diabetes: It's Up to You in the USA

Guess which of 30 developed high-income countries has the greatest prevalence of diabetes? Yes, topping the list is the USA!

That's bad enough—whoever thought that being an American citizen was a risk factor for diabetes?—but that's not the worst part: When it comes to caring for people with diabetes, the US medical care system (if it can be called a system) is near the bottom of the list.

There's a group called the Organization for Economic Cooperation and Development (OECD), consisting of 30 major nations. They churn out a lot of statistics, and, according to the head of its health division, the United States is shortchanging its citizens with diabetes.

Though diabetes can be manageable with proper day-to-day care, serious complications can land people in the hospital. In the United States, according to the OECD health director, hospital admissions for acute complications of diabetes occur at the rate of 57 for every 100,000 people. The average rate for all OECD nations is just 21 admissions. In the Netherlands, it's 8!

Now, this is grisly, but in 2006, there were 36 diabetes-related lower-limb amputations per 100,000 US citizens. The OECD average was just 15; in Austria, 7! Austria has a prevalence of diabetes very nearly the same as the United States, but the US rate of foot and leg amputations is five times higher.

I'm reporting this not to disparage the US health care system but, rather, to emphasize that if you're a Yankee, you live in a nation where you are more likely to develop diabetes and less likely to receive adequate medical treatment or preventive care.

In order to prevent diabetes or avoid serious complications, you have to count on your own initiative. That's what the Diabetes Rescue Diet is all about.

lost more weight than those assigned to the low-fat one—and they saw more improvement in their levels of "good" HDL cholesterol and "bad" triglycerides, too.

The Mediterranean way of eating also improves HbA1c and post-meal blood sugar levels, researchers in Italy found. In a 6-year study, the team examined HbA1c measurements in 901 people with type 2 diabetes who followed a Mediterranean-type diet. To find out how closely these patients stuck to that way of eating, researchers assessed their diets using a 9-point scale—the higher the score, the better the adherence.

By the end of the study, the researchers found that those in the top third of adherence—scores of 6 to 9—had A1c levels 0.9 percent lower than those in the bottom third (zero to 3). This is a huge difference. I was curious to see how these results compared with antidiabetes drugs, so I did some research. It turns out that one popular drug, pioglitazone, also lowers A1c 0.9 percent—same difference!

Researchers also measured blood sugar levels 2 hours after meals, because holding down these spikes is very important for health. The highest-adhering patients had blood sugar spikes nearly 40 milligrams lower than the lowest-adhering patients—a major healthy difference. They also had slimmer waistlines and lower body mass indexes and were less likely to have metabolic syndrome. With all these benefits, it's no wonder that people with diabetes on our diet need a lot fewer drugs!

Deadly Heart Disease Cut 79 Percent!

Among people with diabetes, the most common cause of death is heart disease. In fact, their risk is two to four times higher than that of folks without diabetes and appears earlier in life, is almost as common among women as men, and is more often fatal. The good news is that the Diabetes Rescue Diet is fighting to protect your heart every inch of the way, whether or not you have diabetes.

At the beginning of this chapter, I described a large study conducted in Australia that found that people who eat the most Mediterranean-style foods have a 79 percent lower risk of dying from coronary heart disease. Coronary heart disease is the most common cause of death in

What's HbA1c?

The hemoglobin A1c test—HbA1c, for short—is the gold standard of measuring diabetes control. This blood test, given by your doctor every 3 months, is the "big picture." It's an average of your blood sugar control over a 2- to 3-month period and is teamed with the "snapshots" of everyday home finger-stick blood sugar tests.

Hemoglobin is a substance in red blood cells that carries oxygen throughout your body. When diabetes is not controlled, sugar builds up in the blood and combines with hemoglobin, becoming "glycated."

For people without diabetes, the normal range for the HbA1c test is between 4 and 6 percent. Because studies have repeatedly shown that higher HbA1c levels correlate to a higher risk of developing complications related to diabetes, the goal for people with diabetes is an HbA1c of less than 7 percent.

The good news? Lowering your blood sugar by only 30 points reduces your HbA1c by 1 percent and decreases your risk of long-term problems by 15 to 30 percent. In fact, a study of almost 5,000 people, reported in the *British Medical Journal,* found that each 1 percent reduction in HbA1c reduced, on average, heart attacks by 14 percent, death by 21 percent, and damage to tiny blood vessels (as in the retina of the eye) by 37 percent.

Western countries and includes chest pain, heart attack, and heart failure. That's a lot of protection!

In another study of almost 75,000 female nurses ages 38 to 63, published in the medical journal *Circulation,* researchers examined the association between a Mediterranean style of eating and the risk of coronary heart disease, as well as death from cardiovascular disease, in women. The researchers tracked these women for a long time—20 years. As in other studies that assessed the health benefits of the Mediterranean diet, the researchers used a scoring system of 0 to 9—again, the higher the score, the better the adherence to the diet. The findings were impressive. The women in the top 20 percent had a huge 39 percent lower risk of fatal heart disease and 13 percent lower risk of a deadly stroke, compared with those in the bottom 20 percent.

Men's hearts benefit as well. In a Spanish study of 41,000 men, researchers found a 40 percent lower risk of unstable angina or fatal or nonfatal heart attack in those who stuck mostly to a Mediterranean style of eating (as defined by a questionnaire of more than 600 foods). That's a higher rate of protection than can be obtained by the use of widely prescribed statin drugs, which lowers major coronary events by 31 percent.

I'm not suggesting that the Mediterranean diet is always a better solution than doctor-prescribed statin drugs, but I'd venture to say that if it could be patented and put in a bottle, it would the most profitable medication in history!

If You've Already Had a Heart Attack . . .

A Mediterranean-style diet can *still* save your life. Let's look at the results of the prestigious Lyon Diet Heart Study, which began in 1988 to study whether a Mediterranean diet could reduce the incidence of second heart attacks or heart-related deaths in a group of 605 people who had survived a first heart attack.

On a Mediterranean-style diet versus a "prudent" Western diet (similar to the average American diet, I read), the rate of serious complications fell from 50 to 70 percent. The Mediterranean-style diet was so successful that the researchers called off the trial and switched all the patients over to it!

These findings strongly suggest that it's never too late to protect your heart by doing one simple thing: improving your diet.

Live Longer and Stronger!

While the Diabetes Rescue Diet protects against diabetes and its complications (and more, as you'll see), the ultimate payoff is staying alive. Whether you have diabetes or not, it's good to wake up to enjoy another sunrise, another walk with your dog, another family get-together. And the Diabetes Rescue Diet really does keep you going longer and stronger!

The Low-Fat Diet: Flat-Out Wrong?

Cutting down on fat has long been central to standard diet recommendations. And one of the biggest differences between a Mediterranean-based diet and others is that it is not low but moderate to even high in fat—thanks to olive oil (not bacon cheeseburgers!).

Back in the late 1990s, a huge study was launched to "prove" that a low-fat diet would help prevent heart disease. Heart disease, remember, is the number one immediate health threat if you have diabetes—responsible for 80 percent of all diabetes-related deaths.

Nearly 50,000 women participated at 40 clinical centers. Those who were assigned to the low-fat diet were not simply told to eat less fat—they received "intensive" training in behavioral modification in group and individual sessions. The goal was to reduce fat intake to just 20 percent of daily calories. They were also told to increase their consumption of fruits, vegetables, and grains.

Eight years later, the women who ate low-fat diets and those who simply followed their regular eating style were examined for prevalence of heart disease. Would there be a notable difference in heart disease? Findings:

- Coronary heart disease: no statistically significant difference

- Cardiovascular disease: no statistically significant difference

- Stroke: no statistically significant difference

The researchers also looked for any difference in the rate of invasive breast cancer, as it was thought that a low-fat diet would be protective, but there was nothing there, either. In these pages, you'll read about study after study showing how, in contrast to the failure of the low-fat approach, a Mediterranean-style diet does prevent heart disease—and cancer as well. People with diabetes are at increased risk of both, so this is especially important.

Keep in mind: Though our diet is higher in fat, it's heart-healthy monounsaturated fat—largely from olive oil, as well as nuts, peanut butter, and fatty fish. That could be key: Of the various fats reduced in the low-fat trial, the type of fat most cut was monounsaturated!

A European study of almost 2,500 men and women ages 70 to 90 in 11 countries found major longevity power associated with a Mediterranean-style way of eating. In a 12-year study called Healthy Aging, the team found lower mortality when all four parts of the program were considered—consumption of the foods themselves, regular physical activity, not smoking, and moderate alcohol use. Together, these factors contributed to an astounding 65 percent lower risk of death! To give you an idea of what that means in practical terms, consider findings from some other studies.

In a study of more than 250,000 men and women ages 50 to 71, those who followed an intense exercise program—the kind of workout you get when playing sports—lowered their risk of mortality by 32 percent. In another study of more than 30,000 heart patients, taking the cholesterol-lowering drug pravastatin lowered risk of overall death by 21 percent. While these findings on exercise and cholesterol medication are impressive, they're not even close to the 65 percent reduction found in the Healthy Aging study.

Another study published in the *American Journal of Clinical Nutrition* compared the staying-alive power of a Mediterranean-style diet with the Healthy Diet Indicator of the World Health Organization and a carbohydrate-restricted diet (similar to the popular Atkins diet). This study followed a group of older Swedish men (average age: 71) for 10 years. The Mediterranean-style diet was the only one that extended life, with a 29 percent lower risk of overall death and a 37 percent lower risk of death from heart disease. In contrast, the men who followed a carbohydrate-restricted diet had a 19 percent higher risk of dying during the 10-year follow-up and a scary 44 percent greater risk of dying of cardiovascular disease.

And yes, "eating Mediterranean" boosts the longevity of older Americans, too. Noting that nine separate studies in Europe and Australia showed a protective effect against mortality, an international team of researchers—including several from the United States—set out to see if that was also true among the US population. Following more than 200,000 members of the American Association of Retired Persons for 5 years, the researchers found that a Mediterranean way of eating reduced deaths from all causes—including cardiovascular disease and cancer—by 20 percent in women and 21 percent in men.

Tremendous Protection . . .
without Weight Loss!

Losing weight is linked to a lower risk of diabetes and fewer complications. About 85 percent of people with type 2 diabetes are overweight or obese, so it's no surprise that experts say the best way to protect against the disease is to shed those extra pounds. But the Mediterranean diet delivers tremendous protection without the need for weight loss. So where does that leave the "Lose weight!" commandment?

Well, it's still a good idea if you have or are at risk of diabetes, but it may not be such a good idea to make it your primary means of protection. For most people, weight loss just doesn't work—even when they're enrolled in structured weight-loss programs run by doctors, dietitians, and exercise specialists.

To see if there is some especially fabulous diet that does work, a study carried out at an academic medical center in Boston tried something unusual. They worked with 160 people—all overweight or obese, with at least one other diabetes risk factor: high fasting blood sugar, high blood pressure, or high cholesterol. The researchers divvied up these folks, randomly assigning them to one of four popular diets: Atkins (carbohydrate restricted), the Zone ("balanced" nutrition), Weight Watchers (calorie restricted), and Ornish (low-fat).

After 1 year, the researchers compared the results and later published their findings in the *Journal of the American Medical Association*. Combining results of all four diets, the average weight loss was fewer than 6.5 pounds. That's after a year of dieting! What's more, there was no relationship between which diet people were assigned to and how much weight they lost. The only difference depended on how closely participants adhered to the prescribed plan.

And therein lies the main reason, perhaps, for the weak results: The drop-out rates were huge. Even Weight Watchers, which certainly isn't an extreme diet, had a 65 percent drop-out rate. No diet had less than half the dieters quit before the program was over.

And what benefit did a year's worth of dieting bestow on the health of these diabetes-prone folks? It did improve their cholesterol, but there was no effect on blood pressure and no effect on blood sugar levels. Moral—to me, at least: Being trim is great, but counting on a weight-loss diet alone to give diabetes the slip is not the smartest move you can make.

Terrible at "Dieting"? Perfection Not Required!

One of the best things about the Mediterranean diet is that you needn't follow it perfectly to get great results, as researchers in India—a continent away from the Mediterranean region—discovered.

These scientists wanted to know if the Mediterranean diet would work if modified somewhat for a different culture. They tested that idea in a group of 1,000 patients, all at high risk of coronary heart disease, some with angina and some who'd already had a heart attack. Half of the patients were assigned to a local version of the Step I National Cholesterol Education Program prudent diet, a standard and widely used program. The other half ate an Indo-European diet, which was a localized version of the Mediterranean diet and consisted of more fruits, vegetables, whole grains, legumes, and nuts (walnuts and almonds). Fish and wine were not included, and other vegetable oils, including soy oil, replaced olive oil.

Despite these changes, the Indo-European diet was a major winner against the standard diet. Patients on the Indian-style Mediterranean diet had just half the number of nonfatal heart attacks (21 versus 43) and nearly two-thirds fewer cases of sudden cardiac death (6 versus 16).

These tremendous results suggest that even if you don't follow the Mediterranean diet perfectly, the benefits—at least for controlling heart disease—can be extraordinary. And the better outcome wasn't against just any old diet but against the diet widely prescribed in the United States and other countries.

Remember that heart disease is the single greatest danger to people with diabetes. These unfortunate outcomes were cut in half or more by the Mediterranean diet!

It's Not the Quantity of Your Calories, It's the Quality of Your Food

Research shows that people with type 2 diabetes lose less weight—and lose it more slowly—than people who don't have the condition. There are a variety of reasons why: metabolic problems, other conditions that restrict the ability to be physically active, and weight gain associated with taking insulin or other medications used to treat diabetes, including some pills that are prescribed to control blood sugar.

Even so, experts typically recommend that people lose from 5 to 10 percent of their body weight to reduce the dangers of diabetes. If you weigh 200 pounds, that's 10 to 20 pounds. That's not so much. But according to several studies, losing even that small amount proves tough for people with diabetes.

Baltimore researchers from Loyola College and the Johns Hopkins School of Medicine decided to look at the broad picture of what happens when folks with type 2 diabetes go on "educational and

---

90 Percent of Diabetes Can Be Avoided

The quote below comes from one of the biggest proponents of the traditional Mediterranean diet—a preeminent Harvard nutritionist who has researched the health benefits of this way of eating for almost 2 decades.

> "Together with regular physical activity and not smoking, our analyses suggest that over 80 percent of coronary heart disease, 70 percent of strokes, and 90 percent of diabetes can be avoided by healthy food choices consistent with the traditional Mediterranean diet."
>
> –Walter Willett, MD, chair of the Department of Nutrition at Harvard School of Public Health and professor of medicine at Harvard Medical School

Because the Diabetes Rescue Diet promotes not smoking, as well as regular physical activity, we're talking about the possibility of a 90 percent cut in diabetes risk! If you have diabetes, it's good to know that you can avoid being a casualty of this epidemic—using a knife, a fork, and your own two feet.

---

behavioral interventions"—structured weight-loss programs, led by professionals, that don't involve drugs. They analyzed 18 different trials lasting from 1 to 19 months and found that the average weight loss was 3 pounds.

Really? *Three pounds?*

A clue to the reason it seems so difficult for people with diabetes to slim down comes out of a fascinating study done at the University of Pittsburgh Medical School. Researchers found 12 couples in which both partners were obese, but only one spouse had diabetes, and put them on identical diets for 20 weeks. By the end of the program, the spouses with diabetes had lost only about half as much weight as the nondiabetic ones! The reason for the difference? The people with diabetes simply didn't stick to the diets nearly as well. Lesson learned: It's hard for anyone to lose weight and keep it off, but even harder for someone with diabetes. Again, the Diabetes Rescue Diet is here to save the day!

On this plan, you won't track calories (or fat grams or carbs, either). Although you'll pay heed to eating sensible portions, you won't feel like you're dieting. It makes more sense to prioritize the quality of your diet than simply to try to cut calories.

Oh, and one more thing: The Diabetes Rescue Diet is actually the best way to lose or at least control your weight!

Get Ready to Eat Well and Feel Better

I hope you're convinced that the Diabetes Rescue Diet is simply the best, easiest, and most pleasant way to reduce your risk of diabetes and heart disease and benefit your overall health. The next step is to actually plunge into the plan!

In the next 10 chapters, you'll be introduced to the Rescuers—nine foods that make up the majority of the Mediterranean diet—along with one guideline that is a key component of the traditional Mediterranean diet: eating less meat.

In each chapter in this section, you'll learn about an individual Rescuer and how that delicious item can help you live a full and active life with diabetes, as well as how to best use that food so you maximize its protective qualities. The chapters are stuffed with so many ways to prepare these foods, you'll be digging in before you can say *Salute!* (That's Italian for "To your health!") The Rescuers are:

★ **Whole grains.** Filled with fiber and antioxidants, whole grains— from oatmeal to brown rice—can help steady your blood sugar and lower your blood fats, as well as help you lose weight or keep it off.

★ **Olive oil.** This "liquid gold" is packed with heart-healthy mono- unsaturated fats, and its rich concentration of plant chemicals may help reduce the cellular damage caused by free radicals and help protect "bad" LDL (low-density lipoprotein) choles- terol from oxidation.

★ **Fish.** The omega-3 fats in fish, particularly cold-water fatty fish like salmon, have been found to reduce the system-wide inflammation associated with heart disease and diabetes, as well as lower blood pressure and triglycerides and slow the buildup of plaque in the arteries.

★ **Nuts.** Sweet, crunchy, and delicious, their high content of fiber and unsaturated fats—both monounsaturated and polyunsatu- rated—helps lower total and LDL cholesterol.

★ **Vegetables.** The more colorful, the better! A diet rich in brightly hued veggies—loaded with health-protecting antioxidants and phytochemicals—may lower the risk of type 2 diabetes, heart disease, and stroke.

★ **Beans.** From black beans and chickpeas to pintos and kidney beans, these fiber-packed nuggets are digested slowly, result- ing in a gradual, gentle rise in blood sugar.

★ **Fruits.** Yes, you can eat fruit if you have diabetes! Like veggies, fruits are packed with fiber, vitamins, minerals, and disease- protective phytochemicals.

★ **Red wine and alcohol.** A glass a day will do ya! Moderate con- sumption of alcohol in any form—beer and liquor as well as red wine—has been found to relax blood vessels, reduce blood's ability to clot, and help prevent blood fats from forming the blockages in arteries that can cause heart attack and stroke.

★ **Dairy.** Research points to low-fat dairy as a major diabetes fighter. Low-fat yogurt, cheese, and milk provide all the key nutrients in the full-fat varieties—including protein, calcium, vitamin D, and the powerful antioxidant vitamins A and E—without the saturated fat and cholesterol.

★ **Less meat.** The less red meat (beef, pork, and lamb) you consume, the healthier you tend to be. If you use meat the way you use hot sauce—just a dash—you cut way back on your intake of saturated fat and lower your risk of death from not only diabetes but any cause at all!

While each Rescuer has individual accomplishments, it's when you put them all together that they work their magic. You'll see how it all comes together with the Rescue Meal Plan and Score Sheet on page 144 and more than 80 delicious Rescue Recipes that follow.

But that's not all. In Part 2, Rescue Yourself with Lifestyle, you'll find an easy walking plan as well as a guide on dining out Diabetes Rescue–style. And in Gardening to the Rescue! on page 271, you'll learn how a common pastime in the Mediterranean region can help you be more active and eat healthier. (Anything you grow, you can eat!)

Shortcuts to the Diabetes Rescue on page 300 reveals easy ways to short-circuit your risk of diabetes or manage the condition if you do have it. And in 12 Healthy Bonuses beyond Diabetes Prevention and Management on page 333, you'll discover how the Diabetes Rescue Diet protects against additional health conditions.

You'll begin reaping all the benefits when you turn this page. But there's one last thing you need to know about going Mediterranean: its philosophy of life. Particularly in Italy, France, and Greece, enjoying food and nature is a top priority. I hope this book offers you a taste of that zesty Mediterranean spirit and inspires you to drink deeply of the pleasures life offers—a daily walk, the sun on your back as you work in your garden, a glass of fine wine (if you imbibe)—and, of course, food, glorious food.

Get ready to enjoy a delicious new way of life!

Rescuer No. 1

WHOLE GRAINS

Aim for three to four servings a day

Today for lunch, I got in two servings of whole grains. I didn't eat brown rice, barley, oats, or quinoa, although I enjoy all of these and more. No, my whole grains came from . . . Triscuits. I spread about a dozen of the whole grain rye variety with hummus and *tzatziki*—the creamy, tangy Greek cucumber dip flavored with garlic—and bam: two servings of whole grains down.

   The research is solid: A diet rich in whole grains can help prevent type 2 diabetes and cardiovascular disease. If you already have these conditions, putting a few whole grain servings on the menu each day can help steady your blood sugar, lower your blood fats, and help you lose weight or keep it off.

It's easier to get your whole grains than you might think. Whole grain crackers are one way; popcorn is another. Did you know fresh corn is considered a whole grain, too? And if you're too busy to cook, Uncle Ben has introduced a number of brown rice blends you can prepare quickly.

Plus, there's an array of whole grains with funny-sounding names (see "Catch the Whole Grain Train" on page 28) that can blast you out of a brown rice or oatmeal rut. When it comes to whole grains, you can choose to stick with the familiar or savor new tastes—you just can't lose.

Even better: You don't have to totally give up foods made with white flour, like pasta. Shocked? Don't be. Thanks to the glycemic index (GI), a system that ranks foods by how they affect blood sugar levels, we know that some foods raise blood sugar levels less than others that have the same amount of carbohydrates. Pasta is one of those foods. It has much less effect on glucose than white bread does, even though the two foods' carb content is the same.

Surprised? Good. I like surprising people. In this chapter, I'll explain just why whole grains are a must if you have or are at risk of

---

Get a *Real* Whole Grain Product

Ready to try a whole grain bread or cereal? Shop carefully—labels can be deceiving. To make sure the bread, cereal, or other product you buy is made with whole grains, look at the ingredients list, not the label. The word *whole* should be in front of the word *grain*. For example, "whole wheat flour" describes a whole grain, but "wheat flour" does not. Millet, amaranth, quinoa, and oats are always whole grain, but if you don't see *whole* in front of *wheat, corn, barley,* or *rice*, the grain has been refined.

Products labeled "multigrain," "stone-ground," "100% wheat," "cracked wheat," "seven-grain," or "bran" typically aren't made from whole grains. Color is not an indication of a whole grain, either. Bread can be brown because of other added ingredients.

diabetes, how much of them to eat to protect your health (including your cardiovascular health), and how to prepare them to maximize their power and make them taste great.

What's So Great about (Whole) Grains?

All grains start out "whole," meaning they have three parts: the bran (where most of the fiber is), the germ (where most of the nutrients are), and the endosperm (which makes up the bulk of the seed). They're like tiny jewel boxes packed with nutritional riches like fiber, B vitamins, and minerals, including trace minerals such as selenium, copper, and magnesium. They also contain plant chemicals that research suggests help protect against disease, including diabetes and heart disease.

But the refining process removes the bran and germ. Without these nutrient-dense parts, grains lose 15 key nutrients, fiber included. While manufacturers can and do add back vitamins, minerals, and even fiber, they're fixing what wasn't broken in the first place.

Worse, these fiberless, pulverized grains are digested almost immediately, quickly raising blood sugar to high levels. In response, the pancreas rapidly secretes insulin to ferry that glut of sugar out of the bloodstream. Over time, these blood sugar spikes and the corresponding increases in insulin secretion can lead to diabetes.

Worse yet, soon after you digest these nutrient- and fiber-poor refined grains, your blood sugar crashes, leading to fatigue and hunger . . . often for more empty calories from refined grains (think cookies, cheese puffs, and the like).

Whole grains won't do you like that. Because they retain their bran and germ, whole grains are good sources of fiber, the part of plant foods your body doesn't digest. High-fiber whole grains also help fill you up, so you're less likely to overeat. Plus, a high-fiber diet reduces the risk of diabetes, heart disease, and some cancers.

Whole grains typically have a lower GI, too. Because it takes longer for digestive enzymes to reach the starch inside them, slowing its conversion to sugar, blood sugar and insulin rise slowly and gently.

Whole grains also tend to have a low glycemic load, another tool used to determine blood sugar response. Because it factors in both a

Catch the Whole Grain Train

Ever paired beans with the tiny, nutty-tasting grain called quinoa? Savored the hearty flavor of buckwheat pancakes? Eaten honest-to-goodness rye bread? If not, you're missing out on some really tasty alternatives to better-known whole grains like brown rice, oats, and popcorn.

The next time you're at the health-food store or in the organic section of your local supermarket, investigate these whole grains, their flours, or the foods made with them.

- Amaranth
- Barley
- Buckwheat
- Corn, including whole cornmeal
- Millet
- Oats, including oatmeal

- Quinoa
- Rye
- Wheat, including varieties such as spelt and Kamut and forms such as bulgur, cracked wheat, and wheat berries

food's GI and the actual amount of carbs in one serving, glycemic load offers a more accurate picture of how much a food affects blood sugar. But here's all you really need to know: (1) The lower a food's GI or glycemic load, the less it affects blood sugar and insulin levels; (2) Whole grains generally rank lower on the GI and have a lower glycemic load than refined grains.

White Rice 0, Whole Grains 3

At this point, I must mention the recent findings by researchers in the department of nutrition at the prestigious Harvard School of Public Health, which suggest that whole grains are better than refined ones for people with diabetes (and everyone, actually). These scientists looked at the rice-eating habits of men and women in three studies—the Nurses' Health Studies I and II and the Health Professionals Follow-Up Study. The scientists analyzed questionnaires about diet, lifestyle, and health that the participants filled out every 4 years. In all, the scientists followed almost 200,000 people for a combined 56 years.

Compared with volunteers who ate less than one serving of white rice a month, those who ate five or more servings per week had a 17 percent increased risk of diabetes, after adjusting for age and other risk factors. On the other hand, the participants who ate two or more servings of brown rice a week reduced their diabetes risk by 11 percent, compared with those who ate less than one serving of brown rice a month.

In fact, the scientists figured, replacing just one-third of a typical daily serving of white rice with the same amount of brown would shrink the risk of developing diabetes by 16 percent—and swapping white rice for other whole grains, such as whole wheat and barley, would lower risk by a whopping 36 percent!

The high GI of white rice is likely caused by stripping the bran and germ during the refining process, the study said. It noted, too, that refining also strips away fiber, vitamins, and minerals (including magnesium) and plant chemicals such as lignans, phytoestrogens, and phytic acid, which may help protect against diabetes.

In a 2007 study, scientists analyzed whole grain consumption by crunching data from the Nurses' Health Studies I and II, which tracked the health and dietary habits of 161,737 nurses who were followed for up to 18 years. Compared with nurses who rarely ate whole grains, those who averaged two to three servings a day were 30 percent less likely to have developed type 2 diabetes. When the researchers combined these results with those of several other large studies, they found that eating an extra two servings of whole grains a day reduced the risk of type 2 diabetes by 21 percent.

If you already have diabetes, whole grains come to the rescue again. A 2010 study of women with diabetes, conducted by the Harvard School of Public Health, linked whole grain and bran consumption to reduced overall death rates and cardiovascular disease deaths.

In this latest analysis of data from the Nurses' Health Studies, the researchers followed 7,822 women with type 2 diabetes for 26 years. Periodically, the researchers asked the women to complete food-frequency questionnaires, paying particular attention to whole grains

WHAT IF I DON'T LIKE . . .
WHOLE WHEAT BREAD?

Try sourdough, rye, or pumpernickel. Their hearty, tangy taste may please your palate—and, according to several studies, steady your blood sugar.

Researchers at the University of Guelph in Ontario wanted to know how breads made with different grain flours affected blood sugar both immediately after they were eaten and after a second meal. Once a week for 4 weeks, the researchers had 10 overweight men eat 50 grams of a different type of bread—white, whole wheat, whole wheat barley, or sourdough—both at breakfast and 3 hours later, at lunch (which happened to be 6-inch Subway sandwiches made with white bread, washed down with 10 ounces of orange juice). The researchers tested the men's blood sugar both after breakfast and 15 minutes after lunch.

For both meals, and during the entire study, the sourdough bread produced less of a blood sugar response than the other breads, even whole wheat and whole wheat with barley. Most likely, fermentation in sourdough bread changes the nature of its starches, which has a steadying effect on blood sugar, the researchers said.

Perhaps you like pumpernickel bread, made with coarsely ground rye flour. This hearty, dark-brown bread contains a dynamic duo of diabetes control: acetic acid in its sourdough starter and soluble fiber in its rye flour. Together, these ingredients make pumpernickel's glycemic load lower than that of whole wheat bread (and white bread, too).

In a study on rye bread, researchers at Lund University in Sweden found that people who ate bread made with refined white rye flour (made from the inner white part of the rye kernel) had better blood sugar and insulin control right after a meal than those who ate bread made with a combo of white flour and rye bran.

All of these breads make great sandwiches. Just be sure to read labels before you buy—most rye and pumpernickel breads sold in the States are made mainly of refined wheat flour. One brand to try: Rubschlager cocktail breads. One serving is equal to three mini slices, the perfect amount for a small double-decker club sandwich. The cocktail breads come in sourdough, rye, and pumpernickel.

and their components: cereal fiber, bran, and germ. During the study period, 852 women died of any cause, including 295 who died of cardiovascular disease. The women who ate the most bran had a 35 percent lower risk of death from heart disease and a 28 percent lower risk of death from all causes than women who ate the least bran.

The study also showed that women who ate the most high-fiber grains had a 55 percent lower risk of death from all causes and a 64 percent lower risk of stroke and heart attack than those who ate no whole grains at all.

A Good-Grain Bonus: A Flatter Belly

Carrying some extra pounds right in front? Pumping up the whole grains in your diet may flatten that belly bulge as it lowers your risk of diabetes and cardiovascular disease, recent research suggests.

In a 2010 study, researchers at Tufts University's Jean Mayer USDA Human Nutrition Research Center on Aging analyzed dietary surveys and body-fat scans conducted among more than 2,800 men and women between ages 32 and 83. The researchers factored in smoking history, alcohol consumption, and fruit and veggie intake, among other lifestyle habits. Even so, the participants who reported eating three or more servings of whole grains and less than one serving of refined grains a day had about 10 percent less belly fat, compared with those who reported eating up to four servings of refined grains a day.

The study also found that those who ate an average of three servings of whole grains a day plus four or more servings of refined grains didn't lose their belly rolls. So you can't just add servings of whole grains, this study found—you have to subtract refined grains, too.

In another study conducted in 2008 at Pennsylvania State University, researchers split 50 obese men and women ages 20 to 65 into two groups—one instructed to eat only refined grains and the other to eat only whole grains—and had both of them cut calories for 12 weeks. The folks in both groups had metabolic syndrome, a cluster of risk factors including high blood pressure, unhealthy cholesterol levels,

Go Ahead, Eat Some Pasta

If you want to try whole wheat pasta, that's great. But I promised you could eat regular pasta, and you can, without guilt.

That's right—a half cup of spaghetti or pasta won't blow your blood sugar levels. That's because pasta is made from durum wheat, which your body digests more slowly than it does similar white flours. (You still need other whole grain foods for the phytonutrients that only they can provide.)

Foods with a glycemic index (GI) ranking of under 55 hold blood sugar levels steady. With a GI of 41, spaghetti is a perfectly acceptable indulgence. Macaroni's GI is 45, and fettuccine ranks a surprisingly low 32.

Of course, you'll need to eat one serving of pasta, rather than four or five. Especially when you dine out, be mindful of the large portions restaurants serve. (For more on Rescuing restaurant meals, read the Rescue Eating-Out Guide on page 280.)

At home, don't overcook your pasta. This is crucial. You know how when you overcook noodles or spaghetti, they get mushy? It's because the fiber and carbohydrates have swelled, so the stomach enzymes that break down food can more quickly access the starches and convert them to sugar. And mushy pasta can have a GI ranking of over 60.

Cook pasta until it's al dente, neither too mushy nor too hard. It not only tastes better but also has a lower GI—that nice 45 number. So follow the package directions for cooking al dente. If they're not given, go with the low end of the recommended time (so if the directions say "7 to 9 minutes," make it 7).

and insulin resistance that can develop into cardiovascular disease or diabetes.

Over the 12-week study, both groups received the same dietary advice on weight loss and were encouraged to participate in moderate physical activity. Researchers also asked everyone to eat five servings of fruits and vegetables a day, along with three servings of low-fat dairy products and two servings of lean meat, fish, or poultry.

By the end of the study, both groups had lost weight: The whole grain group lost an average of 8 pounds; the refined grain group, about 11 pounds. Both groups lost body fat, too. But compared with those eating refined grains, those on the whole grain protocol lost significantly more abdominal fat. Plus, their blood levels of C-reactive protein, an inflammatory marker, dropped 38 percent. A high level of marker-reactive protein is thought to place people at a higher risk of diabetes, high blood pressure, and cardiovascular disease. No decrease was found among the refined grain group. Eating refined grains has even been linked to increased levels of C-reactive protein, the study noted, and this most likely canceled out the beneficial effect of weight loss among those participants.

How Much Is Enough?

Experts recommend that adults eat a minimum of three servings of whole grains a day. (I recommend adding an extra serving, if you can.) But it's important to know what "one serving" means. Stick with the single-serving sizes listed below and you'll get your whole grains without overdoing the calories.

- ★ ½ cup cooked grain (brown rice, quinoa, cracked wheat, and so forth)
- ★ ½ cup cooked whole grain pasta
- ★ ½ cup cooked whole grain hot cereal, such as oatmeal
- ★ 1 ounce uncooked whole grain pasta, brown rice, or other grain
- ★ 1 slice whole grain bread
- ★ ½ whole grain English muffin
- ★ 1 cup whole grain ready-to-eat cereal
- ★ 3 cups air-popped popcorn (the mini bags give you the correct amount)
- ★ 5 or 6 whole grain crackers

I recommend spreading out your servings among breakfast, lunch, and dinner. Here are some easy ways to do it. (Check out "Rescued! Five Easy Ways to Get Three a Day" on page 36, too.)

MEET THE
MAXIMIZERS

Irish Oats

Brimming with 4 grams of fiber per cooked cup, this breakfast staple is a diabetes power food. Research shows that oat lovers can lower total and "bad" LDL (low-density lipoprotein) cholesterol and improve insulin resistance. It's all that soluble fiber, a gel-like substance that slows the rate at which your body can break down and absorb carbohydrates, which means your blood sugar levels stay stable.

There's a good chance, however, that the oats in your bowl have been flaked, steamed, rolled, steamed again, and toasted, especially if they're instant. During processing, oats lose their natural taste and texture. To Rescue your oatmeal, I recommend Irish oats.

Also known as steel-cut oats, Irish oats are made when the inner parts of the oat kernel (called the groats) are cut into pieces by steel, then hulled. However, hulling does not strip away the bran and germ, so the oats keep all their nutrients and fiber. In fact, 1 cup of steel-cut oatmeal contains more fiber than a bran muffin.

Compared with instant oatmeal, Irish oats have a lower glycemic index (42 versus 66), which means they won't make your insulin levels spike as high.

Irish oats are a golden color and look a bit like rice. Although it takes 15 to 30 minutes to prepare them, compared with the minute it takes to zap instant oatmeal, you'll be rewarded with their distinctive nutty flavor and pleasantly chewy texture. Tip: To make Irish oats "instant," add ¼ cup oats to ¾ cup water in a bowl deep enough to allow the oats to bubble up without spilling over. Microwave on high for 5 minutes, stir, and nuke for 3 minutes more.

Breakfast is one of the easiest times to get in those servings, especially if you enjoy hot or cold cereal. Pour your whole grain, low- or no-sugar crunchies into a bowl (or nuke your oats or other grain in the microwave), top with low-fat milk and sweet berries, and bam—you're one serving down. Bonus: Eating breakfast is linked to weight maintenance (see Part 3).

Lunch is easy. Enjoy a sandwich made with two slices of whole grain bread or a whole grain pita or wrap. Bam—another two servings under your belt. If you wanted to, you could stop here.

Dinner is a prime opportunity to try a new cooked grain, either alone or fancied up in a healthy pilaf. If stir-fry is on the menu, try serving it over quinoa. It's a great stand-in for brown rice. Or try one of the blended pastas, made with half whole grain flour, half white.

Making the Most of Whole Grains

Fear not—I won't offer the same old suggestions to add barley to homemade soup or whole grain cereal to your yogurt (although I do both, often). There are so many whole grains to try that I'm betting you'll hit upon one you love—hearty buckwheat, sweet Kamut, or maybe tried-and-true brown rice or oatmeal—and brainstorm your own ways to use them. I'll offer some suggestions to get you started.

★ Rip up a slice or two of sourdough bread, and add it to soup or stew.

★ Coat chicken or fish with crushed unsweetened whole grain cereal before baking. (It's a unique way to eat bran cereal.)

★ Make your own oat flour by blending rolled oats in your food processor or blender until smooth. Use for up to half of the flour in pancakes, cookies, muffins, and quick breads.

★ Try kasha (buckwheat groats), which tastes like a heartier, chewier brown rice. My family emigrated from Eastern Europe, so this was a staple on my table. The classic Jewish dish kasha varnishkes teams this grain with fried onions, bow-tie pasta, and chicken or beef stock. To healthy up the recipe, use yolkless egg noodles, onions sautéed in a tiny bit of

Rescued! Five Easy Ways to Get Three a Day

I try to make healthy eating a no-brainer. Once you get into healthy habits, getting in your three or more servings of whole grains isn't tough at all. Here are five ways to do it. Soon you'll be devising your own.

Rescue No. 1

Breakfast: 1 cup prepared oatmeal

Dinner: ½ cup cooked quinoa

Rescue No. 2

Breakfast: 1 whole wheat English muffin

Snack: 1 serving (1 ounce) whole grain crackers

Rescue No. 3

Breakfast: 1½ cups Irish oatmeal

Lunch: 1 (6-inch diameter) whole wheat tortilla

Dinner: ½ cup brown rice

Rescue No. 4

Breakfast: 2 slices whole grain toast

Snack: 3 cups air-popped popcorn

Rescue No. 5

Breakfast: 1 cup whole grain cold cereal

Snack: 1 serving (1 ounce) whole wheat crackers

Dinner: ½ cup tabbouleh

olive oil, and low-sodium stock (if you're on a low-salt diet). Love rice and beans? Substitute quinoa for the white rice—it has a lighter texture that works well with heavier beans.

★ Sprinkle cooked grains such as wheat berries into salads for extra texture and flavor.

★ Try the Middle Eastern dish tabbouleh, made with cracked wheat, lemon juice, parsley, and mint. It's a healthy, tasty alternative to macaroni or potato salad.

★ Try whole grain pasta at least once. It has a denser, slightly nutty flavor that some people enjoy (and it never gets mushy like the kind made with white flour). If you're unsure, try one of the blends that are part whole grain, part white.

★ Snack on air-popped popcorn. A 2008 study found that people who regularly ate popcorn averaged 2½ servings of whole grains per day, while non-popcorn eaters got less than one serving. Shake on a teaspoon of Parmesan (use an actual teaspoon so you don't overdo it), or sprinkle it with a no-calorie sweetener and cinnamon.

★ Or try popped amaranth. Toast 1 tablespoon amaranth seeds at a time in a hot, dry skillet. Continually shake or stir until the seeds pop. Eat as a snack or use them to top soups, salads, and vegetable dishes.

★ Replace one-third of the flour in any recipe with Irish oats (see "Meet the Maximizers: Irish Oats" on page 34) or old-fashioned oats.

★ Add ½ cup cooked bulgur, wild rice, or barley to stuffing (use whole grain bread, too).

★ Use whole wheat pastry flour (rather than regular whole wheat flour) to make lighter, less chewy baked goods.

★ Add ¾ cup uncooked oats for each pound of ground beef or turkey when you make meatballs, burgers, or meat loaf.

★ Make risottos and pilafs with whole grains such as barley, quinoa, bulgur, or millet instead of white rice.

Rescuer No. 2

OLIVE OIL

About 4 tablespoons a day

Without extra-virgin olive oil in my pantry, I'd lose half my regular menu. My wife and I sauté vegetables in it . . . dress our salads with it . . . dip crusty sourdough bread into it . . . drizzle it over a serving of pasta or grilled or steamed veggies . . . and stir it into gazpacho, a tomato-based vegetable soup served cold and often described as a liquid salad. (Yes, I eat a lot of veggies.)

To my way of thinking, I might *eat* without olive oil, but I sure wouldn't have a meal, and I'm sure the citizens of any Mediterranean country would agree. Olive oil's flavor—sometimes fruity, sometimes robust, depending on the variety you select—is rivaled only by its equally wondrous health benefits. No wonder the ancient Greek physician Hippocrates called olive oil the great therapeutic.

In Chapter 1, you read that people with diabetes who ate a Mediterranean diet went longer without blood sugar medication and lost more weight than those on a low-fat diet. In other studies, an olive oil–rich diet has been shown to prevent the accumulation of belly fat—a key factor in the development of metabolic syndrome and full-blown diabetes—as well as improve insulin resistance.

Of course, olive oil's reputation was made on its high content of monounsaturated fat, known to hinder the oxidation of "bad" LDL cholesterol into its artery-clogging form. That's a feat that the artery-clogging saturated fats found in butter, animal fats, and trans fats can't do.

But olive oil's benefits go beyond the monos. Its rich concentration of plant chemicals plays a role as well, recent studies suggest. These potent antioxidants may help reduce the cellular damage caused by free radicals and protect LDL cholesterol from oxidation.

In this chapter, I'll tell you why olive oil is an important part of the Diabetes Rescue Diet, how much of it you need to protect against diabetes and heart disease, and how to enjoy it like Zorba the Greek would.

I recommend spending a few extra bucks and springing for extra-virgin olive oil, derived from the first pressing of the olive and extracted without heat. (You might think of extra-virgin olive oil as "fresh squeezed.") Extra-virgin olive oil is the variety used in many clinical trials and test-tube studies because it contains the highest content of heart-healthy polyphenols. It also boasts the best flavor, which olive oil aficionados typically describe as "fruity," "grassy," "buttery," or "peppery." I just say it's delicious.

The Amazing Belly-Shrinking Oil

There's no doubt that a big belly cranks up diabetes risk. When fat is stored around your internal organs, that fat in and of itself works to block the action of insulin. In fact, much research links belly fat to metabolic syndrome.

MEET THE
MAXIMIZERS
Dark Green Leafies and Olive Oil

Okay, it doesn't have quite the ring of "an apple a day keeps the doctor away." But a daily spinach salad dressed with olive oil may keep the cardiologist at bay.

In a 2011 study, researchers in Florence, Italy, analyzed the food choices of almost 30,000 women over an 8-year period, comparing their eating habits with their risk of heart disease. The women who consumed at least 2 cups of leafy greens or 2½ tablespoons of olive oil each day had the lowest heart disease rates of all—up to 45 percent lower—most likely thanks to the B vitamins, healthy fats, and antioxidant vitamins like C, E, and beta-carotene in these nutrition superstars.

Nutrients in leafy greens and olive oil may help with everything from lowering signs of heart-harming inflammation to preventing plaque buildup in the arteries and guarding against the oxidative damage that contributes to heart disease.

There are other ways to get leafy greens and olive oil into your diet. You can sauté kale or spinach in garlic and olive oil, or add chopped leafy greens or broccoli to your stir-fry. For something completely different, try a tasty kale bruschetta. This recipe makes enough for two: Heat olive oil in a large skillet. Add 1 to 2 cloves chopped garlic and a pinch of red-pepper flakes, if you like. Add ¾ pound chopped kale and sauté until tender. Cover, remove from heat, and keep warm.

Now toast or grill two slices of sourdough bread (for a refresher on sourdough's diabetes benefits, see "What If I Don't Like . . . Whole Wheat Bread?" on page 30) and lightly brush with olive oil. Cut a whole garlic clove in half, rub it over the toast, and discard. Top the toast with the kale and serve.

But might the specific amount of carbs, fat, and protein in your diet—and the type of fat you eat—influence where fat gets deposited on the body, maybe even sending it straight to your belly?

Researchers in Spain suspected that it might. And that's important, because having a big belly is a greater risk factor for diabetes, heart disease, and high blood pressure than having hefty hips and thighs.

In their 2007 study, the researchers had volunteers with a family history of abdominal fat and diabetes eat three different diets. Calories were held constant, but the changing factors were the amount and type of fat and the amount of carbohydrates. For the first 28 days, the diets were enriched with saturated fat. Next, each person followed a 28-day plan with a higher amount of monounsaturated fat. In the third phase, carbohydrates were emphasized.

The researchers studied each diet's impact on the expression of a certain gene that affects adiponectin, a hormone produced and secreted by fat cells. Adiponectin regulates sugar and fat metabolism, improves insulin sensitivity, and has anti-inflammatory effects on the cells lining the blood vessel walls. Low blood levels of adiponectin are common in obesity, a marker for metabolic syndrome, and are linked to an increased risk of heart attack.

Compared with either of the fat-rich diets, the high-carb diet increased the volunteers' belly fat the most, as measured by an enhanced x-ray test. In fact, on the high-carb diet, the volunteers' body fat was redistributed from their legs to their middles, compared with when they consumed the olive oil diet. Ultimately, the diet rich in olive oil bested the diet rich in high saturated fat, preventing not only belly fat accumulation but the insulin resistance and drop in adiponectin seen after the high-carb meals.

Olive Oil Gives High BP the Slip

While you reduce your belly, how about reducing your blood pressure, too? In a 2000 Italian study, people with high blood pressure were able to cut their dosage of blood pressure medicine by almost half—just by swapping other fats for extra-virgin olive oil!

The researchers wanted to study a possible difference in the ability of monounsaturated and polyunsaturated fats to lower blood pressure, so they had 23 people on medication to control high blood pressure follow two different diets that lasted 6 months each. Each diet had the same amount of carbs, protein, and fat: 57 percent carbohydrates, 17 percent protein, and 26 percent fat. For the first 6 months, the volunteers consumed monounsaturated fat in the form of extra-virgin olive oil. For the second 6 months, they received polyunsaturated fats as sunflower oil. The men got 40 grams (about 4 tablespoons) of both oils, and the women got 30 grams (about 3 tablespoons).

The researchers measured these folks' blood pressure every 2 months. After 6 months, the average systolic blood pressure (the top number in a blood pressure reading) in the olive oil group dropped from 134 millimeters of mercury (mm Hg) to 127 mm Hg. In general, for every 10 mm Hg reduction in systolic blood pressure, the risk of any complication related to diabetes drops by 12 percent.

The olive oil group's diastolic pressure (the bottom number) fell, too—from 90 mm Hg to 84 mm Hg. In the sunflower oil group, there was no significant change in either systolic or diastolic blood pressure.

During the study, a separate group of doctors—who did not know which diet the volunteers were following—adjusted the patients' blood pressure medication. The folks on the olive oil diet were able to reduce their daily dosage by a staggering 48 percent, the study found. By contrast, on the sunflower oil diet, medication use dropped by only 4 percent. And during the olive oil phase, eight volunteers were able to control their blood pressure without any medication at all. This didn't happen with the sunflower oil diet.

Olive oil's beneficial effect on blood pressure may even benefit people with diabetes who have high blood pressure, a 2009 study conducted in Spain found. In the 4-week study, researchers fed 40 older people—17 with diabetes and 23 without—a diet rich in virgin olive oil. The team tracked the volunteers' blood pressure as well as their LDL cholesterol, oxidized LDL lipids, and fatty acids.

Systolic blood pressure dropped from 144 mm Hg to 137 mm Hg, the study found, and slightly more (10 mm Hg) in those without diabetes. As a bonus, the virgin olive oil prevented LDL from oxidizing. That's mostly likely due to virgin olive oil's high antioxidant content and because, compared with polyunsaturated fats, monos are less susceptible to oxidation.

Oil Up Your Heart Protection

There's no doubting the link between olive oil consumption and a healthy heart—scores of studies have reached the same conclusion. For example: Men who consumed as much as 2 ounces of olive oil a day chopped their risk of a fatal first heart attack by 82 percent, compared with those who consumed little or none, a Spanish study found.

How impressive is that? Lose 10 to 20 pounds and you'll trim your risk of a first heart attack by 16 percent. Taking low-dose aspirin cuts risk by about 25 percent. So an 82 percent reduction is truly huge!

What about coronary artery disease (CAD), the kind that plugs the arteries that supply the heart with deposits of fat and cholesterol? In a 2007 study of 848 people with CAD and 1,078 healthy people, using olive oil as the only source of dietary fat cut CAD risk by almost half.

In this study, researchers from Greece examined the diets, alcohol intake, physical activity, and smoking habits of all these folks. The researchers also evaluated nutritional habits, including use of oils in daily cooking and food preparation. Even after adjusting for diabetes, high blood pressure, body mass index, and a number of other variables that raise heart disease risk, exclusive use of olive oil

WHAT IF I DON'T LIKE . . .
OLIVE OIL'S DISTINCTIVE TASTE?

I must admit, I can't imagine anyone not liking the taste of extra-virgin olive oil. If you're on the fence about the flavor, I'd encourage you to use it anyway. You can always diminish its flavor by adding the oil to foods like hummus, baba ghannouj, soups, or pizza dough.

If you really don't care for the taste, or if olive oil's too expensive, canola oil is a good substitute. After olive and sunflower oils, canola is the next highest in heart-healthy monounsaturated fats. It also has a neutral flavor and is inexpensive.

was associated with a 47 percent lower likelihood of coronary heart disease. Consuming other fats or oils as well as olive oil, however, conferred no protection.

But monounsaturated fats may not be entirely responsible for high-quality olive oil's protective benefits. Its phenol compounds, shown to be potent antioxidants, may also play a key role. Compared with regular olive oil, the extra-virgin stuff is loaded with these compounds, which research has shown to reduce substances in urine, blood, or saliva that suggest the presence of two heart-threatening processes: inflammation and oxidation.

In a 2010 study of 20 people with metabolic syndrome, Spanish researchers found that olive oil's phenol compounds may "switch off" genes that promote heart-threatening inflammation. During the two-phase study, the volunteers followed the same low-fat, carbohydrate-rich diet—only the breakfasts were different. The first breakfast contained high-phenol virgin olive oil. After a 6-week "washout" period, the participants consumed the other breakfast, made with low-phenol olive oil.

After these meals, the researchers tracked the expression of more than 15,000 human genes in the volunteers' blood cells. Consuming the phenol-rich olive oil switched off 79 genes, many of which have been linked to obesity, high blood-fat levels, diabetes, and heart disease. Further, several of the turned-off genes are known to promote inflammation and so may be involved in "cooling off" the inflammation that accompanies metabolic syndrome.

A Few Drizzles a Day Will Do Ya

Olive oil will always be identified with the Mediterranean diet—healthy, delicious, satisfying, and a pleasure to stick with for life. That said, there's no official guideline on how much olive oil you need to stay healthy.

What we do know is that the Mediterranean diet is comprised of 35 to 40 percent fat—mostly good fats and mostly in the form of olive oil. And for guidance, we can turn to the many clinical studies conducted on the benefits of this way of eating.

In these studies, to reap olive oil's protective effects against diabetes and heart disease, participants typically consumed from 2 to 4 tablespoons a day. But in some studies, they consumed even more. In one case-control study, researchers found that their subjects were taking in an average of 54 grams—about 2 ounces—a day. In one 2010 clinical trial, researchers in Spain had their participants consume a liter a week. That's 4.2 *cups*! I'm not advising that you go that far, but perhaps Americans are too conditioned to keep fat to a minimum.

Let's do the math on 2 ounces a day—a reasonable amount. Two ounces equals 4 tablespoons. A tablespoon of olive oil contains 120 calories, so having 2 ounces would equal 480 calories. That amount is less than 25 percent of a 2,000-calorie diet. Not bad at all.

Of course, you'd have to make sure that you were having 4 tablespoons and not double or triple that amount. If the Greeks and Italians have figured out how many tablespoons to soak up with a piece or two of bread, or how much to dress a salad with or dribble over a serving of pasta, so can you.

A Cheat Sheet for Cooks and Bakers

Sure, you can use olive oil in place of butter or margarine. Use this chart to convert the butter or margarine called for in recipes to olive oil. The conversions work great even in cake and pastry recipes.

FOR THIS MUCH BUTTER OR MARGARINE:	USE THIS MUCH OLIVE OIL:
1 tsp	¾ tsp
1 Tbsp	2¼ tsp
2 Tbsp	1½ Tbsp
¼ cup	3 Tbsp
⅓ cup	¼ cup
½ cup	¼ cup + 2 Tbsp
⅔ cup	½ cup
¾ cup	½ cup + 1 Tbsp
1 cup	¾ cup

That said, I do suggest what many experts on the Mediterranean way of eating have advised—that you substitute olive oil for other fats, especially saturated and trans fats, rather than just add olive oil to your diet. Bear in mind that the idea is to use olive oil as part of your total healthy-fat intake, not in addition to it. So as you reach for the olive oil, remember that a "drizzle" isn't a downpour but more like a tablespoon. Fortunately, olive oil is so flavorful that a couple of table-spoons will be enough.

6 Ways to "Insure" Your Olive Oil

Extra-virgin olive oil isn't cheap, so be smart: Store it properly to extend the potency of its antioxidants and nutrients. Use these tips to protect your precious oil from its sworn enemies—light, heat, and air.

Reach for the back of the shelf. At the grocery store, reach for olive oil that's at the very back of the shelf, where it's been protected from the fluorescent lights.

Buy small quantities. You may be tempted to buy huge, relatively inexpensive tins or jugs because they seem like a bargain. But most olive oils have a shelf life of 18 to 24 months, and, unless you're cooking for an army, you're not likely to use it all up by its expiration date. And if you don't, you'll have a big tin or jug of rancid oil. The best strategy: Choose a tiny container of the best extra-virgin olive oil you can afford. You'll use it up quick, while it's still fresh.

Choose the right container. If your oil comes in a plastic or clear glass bottle, pour it into a container made of tinted glass, ceramic, porcelain, or nonreactive metal such as stainless steel, olive oil experts recommend. Or just buy it in a tin. Don't use containers made of copper or iron, no matter how pretty they are. The chemical reaction between olive oil and metal will damage the oil and may produce toxins. Don't store olive oil in plastic containers, either—the oil can leach harmful substances out of the plastic.

Shield olive oil from light. A bottle of gold-green olive oil in a cut-glass bottle, shining in the sun, looks gorgeous on your windowsill. Problem is, that sunlight is destroying all the heart-healthy components. If your oil is in a clear glass container, wrap the bottle in foil and stow it in a dark cupboard.

Store it away from heat. While it's convenient to keep olive oil near the stove, heat will quickly turn it rancid. The ideal temperature for olive oil is 57°F, so move it from your cooking area to that cool, dark cupboard or your pantry.

Consider keeping it in the fridge. While the oil will get cloudy and solidify, this will not significantly affect its quality or flavor. When you warm the oil to room temperature, it will return to a liquid state, its benefits intact. It'll taste good, too.

A Dozen Ways to Oil Up Your Diet

I've heard that some people rub their Thanksgiving turkey with extra-virgin olive oil instead of butter. What a great idea. Here are some other easy, tasty ways to get your daily drizzles.

★ To keep from using too much oil on your salad, buy a stainless steel (not plastic) plant mister, wash and dry it, then fill it with olive oil. When your greens are in your bowl, give them three or four quick spritzes of oil, then add your vinegar. You'll be surprised at how little oil a salad really needs.

★ If you love the taste of fresh herbs but hate to chop them, try an extra-virgin oil infused with oregano, basil, or garlic.

★ Stir a tablespoon into your favorite soup just before you eat it. It's a quick way to get a serving of olive oil without making a salad.

★ For an easy appetizer, toast baguette slices under the broiler, rub them lightly with a cut clove of garlic, and add a drizzle of olive oil.

★ In the mood for fries? Coat a baking pan with cooking spray. Slice a whole potato into thin strips and place in a bowl. Add 1 tablespoon olive oil and dried rosemary to taste and stir to coat. Place the strips on an ungreased pan and bake at 450°F for about 45 minutes, turning at least once.

★ To make a tasty, heart-healthy dip, drain one can of beans (any kind—many people like white beans). Place in your food processor and add a squeeze of lemon, chopped garlic to taste, and 3 tablespoons olive oil. Process, then season to taste with your favorite herbs, and enjoy with whole grain crackers or bread.

★ Here's an oldie but goodie: Rather than spread bread with butter, dip it into olive oil. You might grate a bit of Parmesan into the oil. Or place a small dish of oregano or thyme next to the oil, and dip the bread into the oil, then the herbs.

★ Mash steamed cauliflower with a tablespoon of olive oil.

★ For the ultimate mashed potatoes, whip together cooked potatoes, roasted garlic, and olive oil and season to taste.

★ Substitute extra-virgin olive oil for other oils in baked goods.

★ Substitute olive oil for butter when you make sauces.

★ Dribble a bit of olive oil over cooked pasta, steamed veggies, or grilled seafood or meat before serving.

Rescuer No. 3

FISH

At least two to three servings (8 ounces total) per week

I grew up near the Jersey shore, so I ate fish a lot. I even caught it myself, surf casting for flounder and sea bass and digging up clams in the surf and eating them raw. I still love fish, especially tuna or salmon sushi, pickled herring, and squid, also known as calamari. (I eat it broiled, though, not battered and fried.) Italians really know their squid. On a hiking trip along the eastern coast of Italy, my wife and I stopped for lunch and were served squid five different ways!

Maybe you're not as fish-crazy as I am. But if you have or are at risk of diabetes, it's smart to make fish a regular part of your diet, as the Greeks, Italians, and other Mediterranean peoples do. First, fish is good for your waistline—it's typically lower in fat than other animal proteins. Second, fish is good for your heart, particularly those species that live in cold waters. These cold-water fish, which include salmon, trout, herring, tuna, sardines, and mackerel, are rich in heart-healthy fats called omega-3 fatty acids. Imagine that—a "fatty" food that's actually good for you.

Fish contain two types of omega-3 fats: EPA and DHA, short for eicosapentaenoic acid and docosahexaenoic acid. (Thank goodness that you only have to eat them, not pronounce them.) Large population-based studies have found that people who eat fish tend to have healthier hearts, and omega-3s from fish have been found to lower blood pressure and triglycerides, slow the buildup of plaque in arteries, reduce the risk of abnormal heartbeats (arrhythmias) that can lead to sudden death, and reduce the system-wide inflammation associated with heart disease and diabetes.

Eating fatty fish has also been shown to pump up "good" HDL cholesterol. For example, a 2009 study from Loma Linda University in California found that participants who ate two servings of salmon a week for just 1 month raised their HDL by 4 percent.

The health benefits of fish are so compelling that federal dietary guidelines, as well as the American Heart Association, recommend eating 8 ounces of fish and seafood a week. Unfortunately, current figures show that we eat less than half that amount, mostly in the form of fried, battered fish or fast-food sandwiches loaded with artery-clogging saturated fat.

But read on, fish skeptics. In this chapter, I'll convince you that fish isn't just good for your heart and blood sugar—it's just plain good. The best part: Fish is quicker and easier to make at home than you might think.

Catch of the Day: Lower Diabetes Risk

No doubt about it, fish is a diabetes-friendly food. As fish consumption rises, diabetes risk falls, studies that have examined the link between a fish-rich diet and diabetes have found. In one Dutch study of 175 men and women, those who ate less than an ounce of fish a day slashed their diabetes risk by 60 percent.

It doesn't much matter what kind of fish you fancy, as long as it's prepared in a healthy way (more on that later). While the health benefits

MEET THE
MAXIMIZERS

Tuna, Salmon, and Mackerel

Sure, you could eat a tuna sandwich a couple of times a week, but then you'd miss out on a crucial part of "going Mediterranean": that each meal is a celebration. The ideas below make it easy to get more of three omega-3 powerhouses into your diet—deliciously.

Canned albacore tuna: Why opt for the same-old same-old sandwich with mayo and diced celery? Here's a tuna salad with a Mediterranean twist: To a 3-ounce can of albacore tuna, add ½ cup cannellini beans, 1 tablespoon feta cheese, and 2 tablespoons olive oil vinaigrette. Enjoy it on whole grain crackers or a satisfying slice of sourdough.

Salmon: Grilled rather than fried, the old-fashioned salmon burger gets a health and flavor makeover: Coat a grill rack with olive oil cooking spray. Preheat your grill to medium-high. Cut ½ pound skinless salmon fillet into 1-inch cubes and pulse in a food processor, just enough to grind coarsely. Transfer to a large bowl and mix in 1 tablespoon each Dijon mustard, fresh ginger (peeled and minced), and fresh chopped cilantro; 1 teaspoon soy sauce; and ½ teaspoon ground coriander. Form into 2 patties and season with salt and pepper to taste. Grill for 4 minutes on each side, turning once. For an added kick, spread salsa on the bottom of whole grain buns.

Mackerel: Known as a bold-tasting fish, mackerel can have a mild, buttery flavor when it's cooked just until the center is flaky. Baked with chickpeas, it's delicious. Preheat the oven to 425°F. Place two 4-ounce mackerel fillets in a baking pan greased with 1 tablespoon olive oil. Heat 1 tablespoon olive oil in a large skillet. Add 1 clove thinly sliced garlic and ¼ teaspoon red-pepper flakes. Cook for 2 minutes, or until the garlic starts to turn golden. Add a 15-ounce can crushed tomatoes and a dash each of ground cumin, chili powder, oregano, and salt. Simmer for 5 minutes, then add ½ cup cooked chickpeas. Pour over the fillets. Bake for 15 to 20 minutes, or until the fish flakes when tested with a fork. Serves 2.

of salmon get lots of well-deserved press, in a 2009 study of more than 20,000 people, whitefish like halibut and sole and oily fish like salmon and tuna came out on top. In this study, researchers from the United Kingdom wanted to know whether regular intake of different fish was linked with a future risk of diabetes. So they examined the fish intake of 21,984 men and women, following them for more than a decade.

A small number of those folks ate no fish at all. But of those who did, about three-quarters ate both whitefish (including cod, haddock, sole, and halibut) and oily fish (such as mackerel, kippers, tuna, salmon, sardines, and herring). About half said they ate fried fish, including that English favorite, fish and chips, and about one-third reported that they ate shellfish. After 10 years of follow-up, 725 people developed diabetes.

Those who said they ate at least one serving of white or oily fish a week had 25 percent less risk of diabetes, the team found. The lower risk remained even when the researchers factored in diabetes risk factors such as obesity, lack of physical activity, and low fruit and veggie consumption. Fried fish didn't affect diabetes risk. It may be that the protein provided by fish helps lower diabetes risk by improving the body's use of insulin, the study said.

If you already have diabetes, regular fish meals will hook you some serious heart protection. In a 2003 study, researchers from Harvard divided 5,103 women with diabetes into five categories according to how often they ate fish. The highest group ate fish five times a week or more; the lowest, less than once a month. Compared with women who rarely ate fish, those who had it once a week slashed their risk by 40 percent. And if they ate it five times a week or more, they reduced their risk by 64 percent!

The Fish/Heart-Health Connection

The evidence is stunning: The more fish you eat, the more protection from heart disease and stroke you reap.

★ In a 2002 Harvard study of 84,688 women, those who ate fish two to four times a week and more than five times a week cut their risk of death from heart disease by 31 percent and 34 percent, respectively, compared with those who ate fish less than once a month.

★ In a 1999 study, researchers from Belgium and Japan examined fish intake and mortality statistics from 36 countries. Their data linked fish consumption with a reduced risk from all-cause coronary heart disease and stroke mortality.

★ A 2004 meta-analysis examined the link between death from heart disease and fish consumption, following more than 222,000 people for an average of 12 years. Eating just one fish meal per week reduced risk by 15 percent. When the researchers classified these people according to fish consumption (less than once a month, one to three times a month, once a week, two to four times a week, and more than five times a week), those in the highest-intake group cut their risk by 40 percent.

Newer studies' findings are no less impressive. For example, taking in a lot of omega-3s from fish seems to protect against obesity-related chronic diseases like diabetes and heart disease, a 2011 study found. Scientists from the Fred Hutchinson Cancer Research Center in Seattle studied the Yup'ik Eskimos of southwestern Alaska. The Yup'ik rate of obesity is similar to that of the general US population, but their prevalence of diabetes is significantly lower—3.3 percent versus 7.7 percent. Plus, their traditional diet includes so much fatty fish that they get an average of 20 times more omega-3s from fish than the average American does.

The researchers measured the blood levels of DHA and EPA in 330 Yupiit, 70 percent of whom were overweight or obese. The volunteers gave blood samples and health information via personal interviews and questionnaires. The researchers also analyzed daily diet, body-fat percentage, blood pressure, and level of physical activity.

In participants with low blood levels of DHA and EPA, obesity strongly increased blood levels of triglycerides and C-reactive protein (CRP), a measure of system-wide inflammation. Both triglycerides and CRP raise the risk of heart disease and, possibly, diabetes, previous studies have shown. But obese volunteers with high blood levels of omega-3s had triglyceride and CRP concentrations no different from people of normal weight. The Eskimos' EPA- and DHA-rich diet may protect them in spite of their girth and may partially explain their low incidence of diabetes, the scientists said.

A Word about Mercury and Fish: Relax

If you're concerned about the mercury levels in fish, which some research has linked with a higher risk of cardiovascular disease, don't be. Mercury exposure from fish wasn't found to boost heart disease risk, according to a 2011 study of nearly 7,000 men and women.

Researchers at Brigham and Women's Hospital and Harvard Medical School evaluated data from two studies that included 173,229 men and women who participated in two landmark studies, the Health Professionals Follow-up Study and the Nurses' Health Studies. Every 2 years, the participants answered questions about their medical history, risk factors, disease, and lifestyle.

The researchers selected 3,427 men and women who did not develop heart disease during 11 years of follow-up and 3,427 who did. Using the participants' toenail clippings—a good indicator of mercury levels because the metal binds to the nail protein—the team evaluated the participants' levels of mercury as well as selenium, a trace nutrient thought to protect against the toxic effects of mercury.

Not only was there no link between mercury and higher cardiovascular disease, the study said, but those with higher mercury levels actually experienced slightly lower heart disease rates, which the team attributed to the other beneficial effects of eating fish. Whether high or low, selenium levels weren't linked to cardiovascular problems, either.

The cautions about consuming fish with higher mercury levels, such as swordfish, tilefish, and king mackerel, among women who are or may become pregnant still stand, the researchers said. Current recommendations are that pregnant or breastfeeding women should avoid these fish entirely and eat no more than 6 ounces of white (albacore) tuna a week. Otherwise, you can take "mercury anxiety" off the table.

8 Is the Magic Number

Just 8 ounces of seafood a week reduces heart-related deaths in people with and without cardiovascular disease, research shows. That's just over an ounce a day—not even the amount in an average tuna sandwich! But that 8 ounces, or two meals' worth, nets you about 250 milligrams per day of EPA and DHA.

Fish and seafood varieties that are higher in EPA and DHA include those cold-water oily fish mentioned earlier, such as salmon, anchovies, sardines, herring, Pacific oysters, trout, and Atlantic and Pacific mackerel. But it's fine to mix up your seafood choices between fish rich in omega-3s and those lower in EPA and DHA. In fact, if you eat a variety of seafood, you'll likely limit the amount of mercury consumed from any one type, experts say.

As a bonus, you'll get to experience the wonderfully different flavors and textures that seafood offers. Go ahead, enjoy that jumbo-shrimp cocktail or lobster dinner. But treat yourself to a range of flavors—from mild or sweet (flounder, orange roughy, or monkfish) to intense (wild catfish or herring).

What you can't do: Order fish at a drive-thru window. When it comes to health, fish that's battered and fried won't cut it. In fact, whether you reap the heart-healthy benefits of fish may depend on how it's prepared, a 2003 study of almost 4,000 older men and women found. Researchers studied how eating different types of fish affected the risk of heart problems caused by narrowed heart arteries (coronary heart disease, or CHD). The study participants who ate tuna or other broiled or baked fish at least three times a week cut their risk of a fatal heart attack in half—they had a 49 percent lower risk of CHD, compared with those who ate fish less than once a month. Fried fish or fish sandwiches didn't lower risk at all.

So order fish steamed, grilled, or broiled, or prepare it that way at home. You might also poach it in red wine or marinate it in the tasty South American marinade called seviche (lime, salt, and seasonings). Or wrap your fish in parchment paper; add fresh herbs, onions, and olives; and bake it so it steams in its own juices. I'm especially fond of this method, called *en papillote*. There are so many healthy ways to cook fish that you won't even miss the high-fat butter and creamy sauces.

How Heart-Healthy Is *Your* Favorite Fish?

Are you a fan of fresh trout or tuna? A sucker for salmon or sardines? Mad for mollusks like oysters and clams? Now you can find out how your favorite fish stacks up, omega-3-wise. The table below, from the 2010 Dietary Guidelines for Americans, lists the EPA and DHA content of common fish and shellfish varieties.

COMMON SEAFOOD VARIETIES	MILLIGRAMS EPA + DHA (PER 4 OZ)
Salmon: Atlantic, chinook, and coho	1,200–2,400
Anchovies, herring, and shad	2,300–2,400
Mackerel: Atlantic and Pacific (not king)	1,350–2,100
Tuna: bluefin and albacore	1,700
Sardines: Atlantic and Pacific	1,100–1,600
Oysters: Pacific	1,550
Shark	1,250
Trout: freshwater	1,000–1,100
Swordfish	1,000
Tilefish: Gulf of Mexico	1,000
Tuna, canned: white (albacore)	1,000
Mussels: blue	900
Salmon: pink and sockeye	700–900
Squid	750
Pollock: Atlantic and walleye	600
Crab: blue, king, snow, queen, and Dungeness	200–550
Mackerel: king	450
Tuna: skipjack and yellowfin	150–350
Flatfish: flounder, plaice, and sole	350
Clams	200–300
Tuna: light canned	150–300
Catfish	100–250
Cod: Atlantic and Pacific	200
Crayfish	200
Haddock and hake	200
Lobster: northern and American	200
Scallops: bay and sea	200
Tilapia	150
Shrimp	100

10 Easy Ways to Go Fish

Like many people, I often order fish when I dine out. But it's almost as easy to cook it at home, especially if you use frozen fillets. Even a can of tuna fish or salmon can be whipped into a healthy, tasty dinner salad or entrée. The tips below will get you started.

★ Make a big bowl of tuna salad—enough to last the week. There's your two servings a week right there! The Tuna Salad Sandwich recipe (page 187) will knock your socks off.

★ If you buy frozen fish, make sure you see "frozen at sea" on the label. Just as veggies are frozen at the peak of their flavor and nutrients, so is fish. And top chefs say that the flavor of fish frozen at sea rivals that of fresh.

Reel In Some Kidney Protection, Too

Kidney disease is a serious complication for people with diabetes. But one small, tasty step—adding fish to your menu twice a week—could reduce that risk by a staggering 80 percent, a 2008 British study of more than 22,000 people found.

Researchers in the United Kingdom studied more than 22,000 middle-aged and older men and women, 517 of whom had diabetes. Using dietary and lifestyle questionnaires, the researchers measured both the participants' fish intake and urinary levels of a certain protein, albumin. The presence of albumin in the urine, called albuminuria, is a sign of kidney damage.

The participants with diabetes who ate less than a serving of fish a week were roughly four times (18 percent) more likely to have large amounts of albumin in their urine, a condition called macroalbuminuria, than those who ate fish twice a week (4 percent), the study found. When kidney disease is caught later, during macroalbuminuria, end-stage renal disease typically follows.

It may be that the unique combination of nutrients in fish enhances blood sugar control and improves blood-fat profiles, which in turn protects the kidneys, the researchers speculated.

WHAT IF I DON'T LIKE . . .
FISH?

Experts agree: It's best to get your omega-3s from fish. But if you won't touch the stuff, ask your doctor if fish oil supplements might be right for you.

The three main forms of omega-3s are EPA and DHA, found in fish and fish oil, and alpha-linolenic acid (ALA), found in plant foods like walnuts, flaxseed, and canola oil. To use omega-3s, the body needs to convert short-chain ALAs to long-chain EPA and DHA, but this process takes awhile. Also, because there's more research on the benefits of EPA and DHA, most experts recommend fish oil capsules.

For people diagnosed with heart disease, the American Heart Association (AHA) recommends 1 gram (1,000 milligrams) of DHA and EPA combined. While the AHA recommends that you get this amount from oily fish, supplements are an option if they're taken under a doctor's care. For high triglycerides, the AHA-recommended dosage of EPA and DHA is 2 to 4 grams per day, again under a doctor's supervision.

While up to 3 grams a day of fish oil is generally considered safe, taking more than that may raise blood sugar, keep blood from clotting, and increase the chance of bleeding, research has found. High doses can also increase levels of "bad" LDL cholesterol in some

★ Keep a bag of frozen fish fillets in your freezer. Thaw them, brush them with olive oil and seasonings, and pop them in the oven for 12 to 15 minutes, depending on their thickness. Or use them to make quick fish tacos: Marinate a fillet in lime juice and spices, bake or broil, break it up, then top with cabbage slaw and wrap in a whole grain tortilla. For 1 cup of slaw, mix 1 cup shredded cabbage with ¼ cup each plain yogurt and sliced green onions.

★ Make *salade niçoise*. I love this Mediterranean classic, which includes romaine lettuce, chunks of tuna, small red potatoes, raw green beans, and hard-cooked eggs dressed in olive oil and people. So if you have a health condition that affects blood's ability to clot, or you take medications that increase risk of bleeding, such as warfarin (Coumadin), aspirin, and clopidogrel (Plavix), don't take fish oil supplements without your doctor's okay.

After you get the green light, follow these tips to ensure you get the most from your fish pills.

- When you choose a fish oil supplement, look for a seal. Companies including USP and NSF analyze supplements for real vitamin level and impurities. The seal on the label lets you know that an independent company has tested the supplement.

- Be aware that the amount of EPA and DHA provided is often only about a third of that listed on the bottle. Check the Nutrition Facts label for the actual amount.

- Take your fish pill with food to reduce the risk of common side effects from fish oil, which include an upset stomach and "fishy burp."

- Store your supplement in the fridge. The fish oil will stay fresher longer.

If you're taking a fish oil supplement and notice that you bruise more easily or bleed excessively, stop taking it and call your health care provider.

vinegar. Anchovies are optional. I like to top my salad with a few capers (omit them if you watch your sodium intake).

★ To fresh or canned tuna, add some white beans and a crunchy veggie like celery or fennel, and dress it with a little lemon juice and olive oil. Simple, healthy, and delicious.

★ Add fresh or canned salmon to your vegetable stir-fry, and serve it over brown rice or another healthy grain like quinoa.

★ If you like battered, fried fish, try this crispy baked option: Whisk together a little fresh lemon or lime juice and some olive oil, or whip an egg white or two. Dip fillets of a mild fish into the dressing or egg, then coat with a crushed, unsweetened whole grain flake cereal to which you've added your favorite seasonings. Bake on a wire rack coated with nonstick cooking spray.

★ If you've never tried sushi or sashimi, now's the time. If you can find sushi made with brown rice, all the better. Sushi or sashimi is the ultimate in healthy fast food—you can pick it up, prepackaged, in any large supermarket.

★ If you're in the mood for Italian, whip up pizza fish. Just coat a mild whitefish (or those frozen fillets, thawed) with a chunky tomato sauce, sprinkle on a bit of low-fat mozzarella or Parmesan cheese and Italian seasonings, and bake.

★ Although people with diabetes can't eat raw oysters, cooked ones are fine. To prepare them, shuck them and scrub the shells. Brush the inside of each shell with olive oil and add a layer of fresh spinach. Dip the oysters into Worcestershire sauce, place two on each shell, and sprinkle with feta or Parmesan cheese. Place on a cookie sheet or shallow pan and broil quickly at 450°F to 500°F, or until the edges of the oysters curl.

Rescuer No. 4

NUTS

About 1.5 ounces (a handful) a day

Fatty foods don't come much fattier than nuts. Most varieties pack 50 percent fat; one, the macadamia, contains 76 percent fat! So why do nuts rank near the top of the "must eat" foods for people with diabetes?

Simple: The fat in nuts is largely unsaturated, which protects against heart disease—and people with diabetes need nuts' primo heart protection. No less than five large epidemiological studies have linked a nut-rich diet with significantly lower rates of heart disease. One scientific review suggested that nuts may be one of the most cardio-protective foods you can eat and estimated that for each ounce eaten weekly, the risk of heart disease death falls more than 8 percent!

It's truly amazing how many nutrients Mother Nature has packed into a food this small. Nuts' fiber and unsaturated fats—both monoun-saturated and polyunsaturated—help lower total and "bad" LDL cho-lesterol. Nuts also contain l-arginine, a precursor to the substance nitric oxide, which helps relax blood vessels and lower blood pressure. And you know the stuff added to margarine and orange juice to lower cholesterol? It's called plant sterols, and nuts are loaded with that, too.

Nuts are also good for your blood sugar. Because they're low in carbs, they don't contribute to the large, health-threatening spikes in blood sugar that can occur after some meals. Reduce these postmeal surges

Nuts Nix Metabolic Syndrome

Can you deal with munching 2 tablespoons of nuts a day and going Mediterranean? If you have metabolic syndrome, it may be worth your while. A 2008 Spanish study found that people with this condition who add nuts to a Mediterranean-style diet are more likely to reverse it.

Researchers compared the effects of two Mediterranean-style diets on metabolic syndrome in 1,224 older men and women. More than 60 percent had metabolic syndrome and displayed classic signs of the condition, including elevated blood pressure, high blood sugar, and abdominal obesity.

The researchers randomly assigned the participants to one of two diet "interventions." One group got about 35 ounces (yes, you read that right) of virgin olive oil a week; the other group, 2 tablespoons of mixed nuts a day. A third group, which served as a control, followed a low-fat diet. All groups were allowed to eat as much they wanted.

Among the group that added nuts, the incidence of metabolic syndrome fell about 14 percent within a year, as opposed to a 7 percent decline in those who added olive oil and a 2 percent decline in the low-fat group. Researchers believe that the fiber, potassium, magnesium, calcium, and omega-3 fatty acids in nuts help regulate insulin, blood pressure, and inflammation.

A bit more about magnesium: This mineral appears to play a key role in blood sugar balance and insulin function, and several studies have linked higher intakes of magnesium with lower risk of metabolic syndrome.

and you protect against diabetes and cardiovascular disease. That's why most days, I munch an ounce of mixed nuts before lunch or dinner.

All this, and these fat-packed treats may actually help you stave off weight gain. Several studies have associated two or more servings of nuts a week with lower weight and avoidance of weight gain. For example, in a 2010 study, researchers at Beth Israel Deaconess Medical Center in Boston reported that people who ate walnuts at breakfast felt fuller, which made it easier for them to eat less at lunch.

Peanuts may even flatten your belly. (Though technically a legume, the peanut has a similar nutrition profile to other nuts, so for our purposes, consider it a nut.) In a 2009 Scandinavian study, researchers had a group of 25 men and women eat a certain amount of either peanuts or candy for 14 days. For every 2 pounds of their body weight, the participants consumed 20 calories in either candy or peanuts. So someone who weighed 160 pounds ate about 1,600 extra calories over the 2-week period.

When they ate the candy, they gained weight and their bellies expanded in 2 weeks. When they ate the peanuts . . . nothing happened. No weight gain, no belly expansion. Another difference: The peanut eaters exhibited an improvement in metabolic rate—they actually burned more calories! So they got to eat a delicious snack and the calories went up in smoke.

The only downside to nuts is that they're so darn good, it's easy to get carried away. Fortunately, because they're so satisfying, you can indulge in a handful (or a couple of tablespoons of peanut butter) every day. In this chapter, I'll explain why they're a go-to food if you want to prevent or manage diabetes, and how to prepare them to maximize their power and make them taste great.

Say "Nuts!" to Diabetes

Eat fatty nuts almost every day and reduce your diabetes risk—without packing on pounds? Yes, a Harvard study of almost 84,000 women found you can do that. The research team evaluated the link between eating nuts and peanut butter and diabetes risk. Those who ate either food five or more times a week cut their chances of diabetes

Almonds Work Overtime to Help Diabetes

Almonds are known as a very healthy food—packed with fiber, healthy fats, and more. But if you have diabetes, they have an exclusive benefit for you—a big one!

In a recent report from Arizona State University, researchers gave some people almonds to eat before a bagel meal (rich in carbs), while others got the same meal without almonds.

In people who had diabetes, the almond addition reduced postmeal blood sugar rise by a very impressive 30 percent. The other people experienced no such effect.

Flattening after-meal blood sugar spikes is very important for people with diabetes. The authors point out that 50 to 70 percent of all daylong high blood sugar comes from these after-meal rises. Plus, high spikes have been closely linked to increased heart disease.

A special group ate almonds not just before a few meal, but every day for 12 weeks. Their A1c blood sugar counts went down 0.3 percent, making almonds comparable to the prescription drug acarbose, which reduces A1c by about 0.4 percent, according to the researchers.

Other studies have found benefits from almonds but with unrealistically high amounts. The great thing about this new study is the small amount used—just 1 ounce!

by 27 percent, compared with those who rarely or never ate them; it's possible the healthy fats increase insulin sensitivity. Better still: If they were at a healthy weight, the frequent nut eaters slashed their risk by 45 percent. These lower risks held up, even after researchers controlled for factors known to raise diabetes risk, including being overweight, having a family history of diabetes, and doing too little physical activity. Best of all: Nut intake wasn't associated with weight gain.

Already have diabetes? Nuts to you, too! Just an ounce of any type or a tablespoon of peanut butter most days of the week may slash your risk of heart disease nearly in half, a 2009 study of more than 6,000 women with type 2 diabetes found. To examine the link between nut intake and cardiovascular disease, these researchers, also from Harvard, analyzed the results of diet questionnaires that 6,309 women with diabetes completed every few years between 1980 and 2002. In that time, 634 women experienced strokes or coronary "events," including heart attacks.

The women who ate at least five servings a week of nuts or peanut butter (a serving equals an ounce of nuts or a tablespoon of peanut butter) had a 44 percent lower risk of heart disease and events such as heart attack or stroke, the study found. What's more, the frequent nut eaters also had lower levels of total and LDL cholesterol and lower levels of apolipoprotein B-100 (APOB). High APOB levels are associated with the formation of the fatty plaques that cause atherosclerosis.

A nut-rich diet's heart-healthy benefits may go beyond cholesterol levels, the study said—it may cool system-wide inflammation, reduce the oxidation of LDL cholesterol, or protect against insulin resistance. By the way, the researchers controlled for dietary factors known to reduce cardiovascular risk, like fat and fiber content, and glycemic load. Even with these factors removed from the analysis, the risk reduction held. This suggests that these nutrients don't completely explain nuts' protective effects, the researchers said. Substances in nuts and peanut butter that are less understood, like phytosterols and arginine, may also be protective.

And if you have prediabetes, you might want to munch almonds. These tasty nuts appear to ward off insulin resistance, a red flag for diabetes, a 2010 study found. When 65 people with prediabetes ate 2 ounces of almonds (about two handfuls) every day for 16 weeks, their fasting insulin levels dropped 23 percent, while those who said no to nuts saw a 19 percent increase. The researchers credited oleic acid, a fat that triggers the release of GLP-1, a peptide that can improve insulin sensitivity.

Nuts: To Your Heart's Content

Many large and well-respected studies have linked consumption of all kinds of nuts to heart health. The first study to show this—the venerable Adventists Health Study—followed 34,000 Seventh-Day Adventists over 12 years. Even in this mostly vegetarian population, those who ate nuts at least five times a week cut their risk of dying from heart disease by 48 percent and their risk of a nonfatal heart attack by 51 percent, compared with those who ate nuts less than once a week.

In the 14-year Nurses' Health Studies, which followed more than 86,000 women, those who ate more than 5 ounces of nuts a week slashed their risk of heart disease by 35 percent, compared with those who ate them less than once a month. And in the 17-year Physicians' Health Study of more than 21,000 men, those who ate nuts at least twice a week reduced their risk of sudden cardiac death by 53 percent, compared with those who rarely ate nuts.

More recent studies back up older findings. In one 2010 analysis of data from 84,136 women, those who ate a daily serving of nuts lowered their risk of heart disease by 30 percent, compared with those who ate one serving of red meat a day.

So pick a nut, any nut. Chances are, your favorite has been found to benefit cardiovascular health.

- ★ **Pistachios.** Pennsylvania State University researchers found that adults who got 20 percent of their calories from pistachios (that's about ½ cup for an 1,800-calorie diet) reduced LDL cholesterol by 12 percent.

- ★ **Peanut butter.** A recent study found that insulin-resistant adults who ate a diet high in monounsaturated fat, like that in peanut butter, had less belly fat than people who ate more carbohydrates or saturated fat.

- ★ **Almonds.** One study found that a heart-healthy diet that included almonds lowered LDL cholesterol as much as a statin drug did. Almonds are also a great snack when you're trying to lose weight. In one study, women who ate almonds had higher levels of cholecystokinin, a hormone that suppresses hunger. In another, of 65 men and women following a low-calorie diet, California researchers found that those who noshed on nuts shrank their waistlines nearly 50 percent more than dieters who didn't, despite consuming the same number of calories. (See "Almonds Work Overtime to Help Diabetes" on page 64.)

- ★ **Walnuts.** Among nuts, they alone are high in omega-3s and may help clear plaque from your arteries. Researchers in Spain

MEET THE
MAXIMIZERS

Walnuts

Richer in heart-healthy omega-3s than salmon, loaded with more anti-inflammatory polyphenols than red wine, and packing half as much protein as chicken, the walnut is a powerhouse of nutrition. A serving of walnuts—about 1 ounce, or seven whole nuts—is all it takes to reap their health benefits.

In fact, a 2010 study led by a researcher at the University of Scranton in Pennsylvania found that walnuts pack almost twice as many antioxidant polyphenols as almonds, peanuts, pistachios, hazelnuts, Brazil nuts, cashews, macadamias, and pecans. These compounds stabilize free radicals—harmful charged particles produced from reactions in our body. When they collide with cells, free radicals can start a chain chemical reaction that can damage or kill those cells.

What's more, the study found, the antioxidants in walnuts are up to 15 times as potent as they are in vitamin E, a powerful antioxidant in its own right. Even the vitamin E in walnuts is special. Walnuts provide a high level of vitamin E in its gamma-tocopherol form, which has been found to provide significant protection from heart problems.

Walnuts also contain alpha-linoleic acid (ALA). The plant version of the omega-3 fats in fish, ALA has been found to dissolve blood clots that can cause heart attack or stroke and protect against dangerous heart arrhythmias.

About 90 percent of the phenols in walnuts reside in the thin, flaky "skin," including key phenolic acids, tannins, and flavonoids. While the skin has a slightly dry, astringent taste, which causes some people to remove it, I say at least try it—that's where the benefits are.

There's another advantage in choosing walnuts. The heat from roasting nuts generally reduces the quality of the antioxidants. People usually eat walnuts raw or unroasted and thus get their full effectiveness.

gave two groups of people a heart-healthy diet that differed in just one respect: One diet included 8 to 13 walnuts a day. After 4 weeks, the walnut eaters had 64 percent stronger artery-pumping action and 20 percent less gunky molecules that initiate atherosclerotic plaque.

Get the Most from Nuts

So just how nuts should you go? Take your cue from the large studies, most of which find that about a handful (1.5 ounces) a day reduces the risk of diabetes and heart disease. Here's what 1 ounce of nuts actually looks like.

- ★ 35 peanuts
- ★ 24 almonds
- ★ 18 medium cashews
- ★ 15 pecan halves
- ★ 14 English walnut halves
- ★ 12 hazelnuts, filberts, or macadamia nuts
- ★ 8 medium Brazil nuts

But why eat only one kind at a time, when there are so many varieties that are so good for you? Mix 'em up. And keep them in your car, desk, or bag—they make delicious, satisfying snacks, and they're easy to eat on the go.

Eating nuts without reducing your intake of saturated fats won't do your heart or waistline any good, so incorporate nuts into your diet sensibly. You'll find lots of easy, unique ideas ahead. But here are five ways to get the most out of those luscious servings.

- ★ Eat the skins of nuts, particularly almonds and walnuts, to get the most antioxidants they have to offer.
- ★ Choose nuts in the shell and you'll probably eat fewer, since it takes time to crack them.
- ★ Swap nuts roasted in oil and dosed with salt for unsalted, raw, or dry-roasted varieties. (Check the ingredients label.) Nuts are often roasted in hydrogenated or partially hydrogenated vegetable oil, which introduces cholesterol-raising trans fats.
- ★ To enhance the flavor of raw nuts, toast them: Spread them on a tray and bake at very low heat—160° to 170°F—for 15 to

20 minutes. This quick process enhances nuts' flavor but preserves their healthy oils. They burn quickly toward the end, so keep an eye on them.

★ Store nuts correctly. To keep them fresh, store them in an airtight container in the refrigerator for up to 4 months. (Nuts can be frozen, too—up to 6 months.) If you buy nuts in the shell, select ones free of cracks and holes. And the heavier nuts are, the better—that heft suggests a fresh, meaty kernel.

WHAT IF I DON'T LIKE . . .
NUTS?

Then don't eat them. Instead, might I suggest a classic American entrée: the peanut butter and jelly sandwich.

Thought your high blood sugar took this childhood favorite off the table? Think again. Numerous studies have found that peanut butter is both heart-healthy and easy on blood sugar and insulin levels. Here's the play-by-play to the perfect PB&J, which contains roughly 400 calories. Two PB&Js a week will bring you close to the five weekly servings of nuts or peanut butter shown to reduce heart disease and diabetes risk.

Step 1: Bring on the bread (160 to 200 calories). Pick a whole grain variety with at least 3 grams of blood sugar–blunting fiber. I love Food for Life's sprouted whole grain sesame bread. Or toast a slice of pumpernickel or sourdough, varieties that have been shown to lead to better blood sugar and insulin levels, compared with white bread.

Step 2: Slather on 2 tablespoons of peanut butter (180 calories). While fat and calorie counts of most brands of peanut butter are similar, all-natural brands contain about half as much sugar as commercial brands. They tend to have less salt, too.

Step 3: Top with jelly (zero to 20 calories). Opt for no- or low-sugar brands—they actually taste fruitier than the sugar-filled cheap varieties. Walden Farms offers a delicious sugar-free strawberry fruit spread. And Smucker's low-sugar preserves (choose from strawberry, grape, raspberry, apricot, or orange marmalade) contain 50 percent less sugar and calories than regular jams.

10 Ways to Go Nuts

By all means, top your salad with slivered almonds or stir your favorite chopped nuts into yogurt or a stir-fry. But there are other ways to bring nuts into your everyday diet. Make sure to get walnuts in there, too. I've been eating a handful of nuts a day for a couple of years, and I recently added walnuts to the mix when I read about how healthy they are. Delicious, too—I actually like the "bite" of that flaky skin.

★ Stir an ounce of chopped walnuts or almonds into your hot or cold whole grain cereal. Walnuts are especially tasty in steel-cut oatmeal, with a little cut-up banana.

★ Make your own snack mix. Preheat the oven to 325°F. Coat a large baking sheet with cooking spray. In a large bowl, whisk together 1 tablespoon olive oil, 1/3 tablespoon soy sauce, and 1/4 teaspoon each garlic powder and ground ginger. Add 1 cup whole grain cereal squares, 1 cup air-popped popcorn, and 2/3 cup peanuts and toss to coat evenly. Spread on the sheet. Bake for 15 minutes, stirring occasionally, until the cereal is very crisp. Remove from the oven and let cool completely, then store in an airtight container. For a spicy kick, use wasabi-coated peanuts, but add them after baking. A 2/3-cup serving of the mix contains 227 calories.

★ Go nuts with your smoothie! In a blender, combine a cup of 1% milk or almond milk, 3/4 cup low-fat yogurt, 1/2 cup sliced strawberries or other fruit, and 2 tablespoons chopped walnuts. Add ground cinnamon and/or sugar substitute to taste and blend for 15 seconds.

★ Add walnuts to your favorite poultry stuffing recipe.

★ Puree walnuts, cooked lentils, and your favorite herbs and spices in a food processor. Add enough olive or flax oil to achieve a diplike consistency.

★ If you love peanut butter, great! If you're looking for a new taste, try almond butter—it has a sweeter, more delicate flavor and is delicious on toast or celery stalks.

★ Make a great pesto for pasta with pistachios. Grind the nuts in a food processor, then blend with fresh herbs, Parmesan, and a little olive oil.

Surprise: Eat Nuts, Weigh Less

Although nuts are high in fat, eating them does not lead to weight gain. In fact, research suggests that they may help people manage their weight better. For instance, in a 2007 Spanish study of 8,865 people, those who ate nuts at least twice a week were less likely to gain weight over a period of more than 2 years than those who never or rarely ate them.

Even when people add nuts to their usual diets, they don't seem to gain. In a small 2007 study from Purdue University, women added 344 calories' worth of almonds a day to their diets and neither ate less nor exercised more. After 10 weeks, they hadn't gained weight. But there's nothing magical about almonds keeping off weight. Studies on walnuts and peanuts have produced similar findings.

The bottom line, according to a 2007 scientific review of nuts and body weight: When added freely to a diet, nuts cause less weight gain than would be predicted, and when added to a calorie-controlled diet, they don't cause weight gain and may make weight loss easier.

How can indulging in such a fat-rich treat not pack on pounds? Researchers think that the fiber and protein in nuts help make you feel full longer, so you're not as hungry and eat less at your next meal. And there's some evidence that nuts may affect metabolism in a way that compensates for their high number of calories.

★ Nut-crusted fish or chicken is delicious. Crush 2 tablespoons macadamia nuts. Dip one 3-ounce portion of chicken breast or 4-ounce piece of fish in 1% milk, then press into the crushed nut coating to adhere. Bake at 350°F for 10 to 20 minutes, or until done.

★ Sprinkle chopped hazelnuts, walnuts, or almonds onto ice cream.

★ Splurge on some of those chocolate-dusted nuts, like Emerald Cocoa Roast Almonds. At 150 calories, 3 grams of fiber, and 1 gram of sugar per ¼ cup, you get the taste of indulgence with all the nutrition of nuts.

Rescuer No. 5

VEGETABLES

Five servings a day

Yes, vegetables brim with fiber, vitamins, and minerals your body needs for peak health. But those nutrients are only part of why they're good for you.

Recent research has revealed that veggies also pack special nutrients and chemicals that slow aging, protect the heart, and help prevent and manage diabetes. These substances, called antioxidants and phytochemicals, are a major reason that a healthy, veggie-rich diet may lower the risk of type 2 diabetes and two of its major complications—heart disease and stroke.

Antioxidants—such as vitamins A, E, and C, beta-carotene, and the trace mineral selenium—protect against oxidation, a natural but damaging process in the body. As you breathe and your cells produce energy, your body constantly reacts with oxygen. This natural metabolic activity produces free radicals—highly reactive molecules that damage cells' proteins, membranes, and genes. Research implicates this "oxidative stress" on cells as the primary cause of aging and many diseases, including type 2 diabetes and heart disease. Antioxidants help protect cells against the effects of free radicals.

Phytochemicals are the substances that put the red in tomatoes, the green in greens, the yellow and orange in carrots and bell peppers, and the purple in eggplant. As it turns out, lots of phytochemicals are also powerful antioxidants. But not all phytochemicals add color. For example, sweet, juicy oyster mushrooms—found alongside common button mushrooms at the supermarket—contain ergothioneine, found to help control blood sugar and cholesterol in people with diabetes and protect against cardiovascular disease.

Of course, not everyone likes veggies. If you do, great—the Diabetes Rescue Diet will be a cinch. If you don't, don't fret. You may not be a vegetable person now, but on this plan, you'll become one. Don't like salads? You'll learn to do salad Mediterranean style. Hate steamed veggies? You'll learn to grill or roast them. Can't eat broccoli unless it's covered in cheese? You'll learn to eat it *Italiano*. In short, you'll experience a veritable veggie renaissance. You'll eat so many types, so many ways, that you'll become an honorary Greek or Italian.

Eating your veggies is like walking for exercise. Once you start, it's so good, you wonder why it took you so long. Before long, you'll eat them not just to prevent or manage diabetes or avoid its complications, but because you actually like them.

Veggies Crunch Diabetes Risk

Study after study suggests that a veggie-rich diet lowers the risk of type 2 diabetes. In one 2008 study of 64,191 Chinese women, it was almost 30 percent lower!

Researchers from the Shanghai Cancer Institute and the Vanderbilt Epidemiology Center in Nashville used food questionnaires the women filled out at the study's start and finish. In the 4.6 years the researchers followed these women's dietary habits, 1,608 developed type 2 diabetes.

Compared with those who ate the lowest amounts of veggies (121 grams per day, or about 4 ounces), those who ate the highest amounts (428 grams per day, around 15 ounces) of yellow vegetables, garlic and onions, tomatoes, broccoli, and green leafy vegetables reduced their diabetes risk by a hefty 28 percent!

Interestingly, in a 2007 analysis of five studies involving 167,128 people, those who ate three or more servings of veggies and fruits a day did not significantly reduce their diabetes risk. But hold on. There's more.

This review also analyzed an additional nine studies of 139,793 people, which examined the relationship between veggie, fruit, and antioxidant intake and diabetes risk. People who had the highest intake of vitamins C and E, flavonoids, and carotenoids—which suggests a diet rich in fruits and veggies—slashed their diabetes risk by 13 percent. The researchers attributed that effect mainly to vitamin E. This vitamin, a potent antioxidant, protects against inflammation, a major risk factor for diabetes. E has also been found to improve the action of insulin, possibly by protecting the insulin-producing cells in the pancreas from free radical damage.

Carotenoids—the pigments that give carrots, orange bell peppers, and sweet potatoes their orange hue—are also linked to a lower likelihood of developing diabetes. In a 2008 study, French researchers examined the diets of more than 1,300 people ages 59 to 71 over a 9-year period. Compared with those with the lowest levels of carotenoids in their blood, those with the highest amounts had a whopping 58 percent lower risk of diabetes. That's even after researchers factored in weight, history of cardiovascular disease, blood pressure, and abnormal levels of HDL and LDL.

If you already have diabetes, get to know mushrooms—specifically oyster mushrooms and maitake mushrooms. Small clinical studies suggest that they may help lower blood sugar in people with diabetes.

For example, in traditional Indian medicine, the mild-flavored,

MEET THE
MAXIMIZERS

Leafy Greens

As diabetes busters, green leafy vegetables are standouts, recent research suggests. In a 2010 British review, eating more of them, in particular, significantly cut the risk of developing diabetes.

Researchers crunched the data in six studies that looked at the links between diabetes and consumption of fruits and vegetables, which included more than 200,000 people ages 30 to 74 in the United States, China, and Finland. Each of these studies followed their participants over periods of 4.5 to 23 years, tracking how many servings of fruits and vegetables they ate each day, then examining who developed type 2 diabetes. The incredible finding: Just over one serving (1.15) of green leafies a day lowered diabetes risk by an average of 14 percent!

Leafy green vegetables seem to protect against diabetes because they contain rich amounts of antioxidants, fiber, and magnesium, studies suggest. They also pack high amounts of polyphenols and vitamin C, both of which have antioxidant properties. That's great news, because there are many different greens to choose from—leafy types like spinach, Swiss chard, kale, and mustard greens; and cruciferous veggies like broccoli, Brussels sprouts, cabbage, cauliflower, and even the Chinese veggie bok choy.

Kale is one of my favorites. I like it Greek style: In a skillet, combine 2 tablespoons chopped red onion, 1 tablespoon extra-virgin olive oil, ¼ teaspoon dried oregano, and salt to taste. Sauté over medium heat for 3 minutes, or until softened. Add 1½ cups chopped kale and stir to coat with the oil and seasonings. Cover the pan and cook for 1 to 2 minutes, or until the kale is wilted. Stir in a pinch of red-pepper flakes, sprinkle with 1 tablespoon feta cheese, and enjoy.

juicy oyster mushroom—excellent in salads and stir-fries—has long been used as an antidiabetes drug. In a 2010 study, researchers from India divided 120 people with type 2 diabetes into three groups and fed them biscuits as part of their diets. Group 1 received regular biscuits. Group 2 got biscuits to which a powdered, standardized extract of oyster mushroom was added. Group 3's biscuits were made with the mushrooms only. The dietitian who gave out the biscuits didn't know which group was getting which biscuit. Only the researchers did.

After 3 months, the researchers found that the fasting blood sugar levels of the two groups that got the special biscuits had dropped more than 100 points—from 225 mg/dL to 113 mg/dL (mushroom added) and from 213 mg/dL to 112 mg/dL (straight 'shrooms). Their HbA1c levels also dropped—from 8.4 to 7.2 percent in the mushroom-added group and from 8 to 6.9 in the group that ate the straight-mushroom biscuits. What's more, their total cholesterol and triglycerides dropped significantly, and their "good" HDL cholesterol levels actually increased. The group that got regular biscuits experienced none of these benefits.

Veggies ♥ the Heart

The more veggies you eat, the better your heart likes it. That's the finding of many well-designed, respected studies.

One of the most recent, published in 2011, examined the effect of veggie and fruit intake on ischemic heart disease. The result of narrowed heart arteries, ischemic heart disease can cause chest pain and lead to heart attack.

For this study, English researchers analyzed data from more than 300,000 people from eight European countries. These folks were from 40 to 85 years old, and their health was tracked for 8.5 years, on average. In that time, 1,636 people died from ischemic heart disease. But those who ate at least eight daily portions of fruits and vegetables were 22 percent less likely to die from the condition, compared with those who ate fewer than three portions a day, the study found.

In this study, one portion was 80 grams (about 3 ounces). Each portion above the lowest intake of two portions reduced the risk of death an additional 4 percent. So if you ate five portions of fruits and vegetables a day, your risk would be 4 percent lower compared with four portions a day, and so on. This newest study underscores similar findings from older studies on other conditions.

Heart attack/stroke. In a 2004 study of 109,635 men and women, Harvard researchers followed the participants' health and dietary habits for 14 years. Compared with those in the category of lowest fruit and veggie intake—less than 1.5 servings a day—those who averaged eight or more servings a day were 28 percent less likely to have had a heart attack or stroke.

Green leafies were the standouts in this study—a single serving

---

Broccoli Boots Diabetes Damage

Blood vessel damage is one of the biggest health problems caused by type 2 diabetes. It's the reason why many who have it have problems with circulation and why they have a higher risk of heart attack and stroke. The main problem: The high blood sugar in those with type 2 diabetes can triple their levels of free radicals—unstable molecules that damage healthy cells, including the ones that line arteries and veins.

Fortunately, those tiny green trees could reverse the damage diabetes wreaks on the heart's blood vessels, a 2008 study suggests. Broccoli's rep as a star diabetes-fighter may hinge on sulforaphane, a compound in broccoli and other cruciferous vegetables that encourages the production of enzymes that protect the blood vessels.

Researchers in the United Kingdom looked at the linings of human blood vessels damaged by high blood sugar levels under laboratory conditions. They found that sulforaphane reduced the production of these cell-damaging molecules by 73 percent.

People with diabetes are up to five times more likely to develop cardiovascular diseases such as heart attack and stroke; both are linked to damaged blood vessels. Broccoli has previously been linked to a lower risk of heart attack and stroke, as have other vegetables of the *Brassica* genus, such as cauliflower, Brussels sprouts, and cabbage.

lowered the risk of cardiovascular disease by 11 percent. The researchers credited these veggies' heart-protective nutrients, which include potassium, flavonoids (phytochemicals found in many veggies and fruits), and diallyl sulfides (found in garlic and onions).

In a 2006 study published in the medical journal *Lancet*, people who consumed more than five servings a day lowered their risk of stroke by 26 percent, compared with those who ate less than three servings a day. In a 1999 study of 114,279 men and women, cruciferous veggies like broccoli offered the most protection against stroke— one serving a day lowered risk by 32 percent.

High blood pressure. Yes, Mediterraneans get it, too—but again, veggies come to the rescue. In a study of 4,393 people from Mediterranean countries, those who ate the most vegetables had a 42 percent lower risk of having undiagnosed blood pressure, a Spanish study found. Those who consumed the most vegetables *and* fruits had a 77 percent lower risk, compared with those who ate the least.

Potatoes, Diabetes Style

While spuds are a part of the traditional Mediterranean diet, evidence suggests that a once-a-week splurge is plenty, especially if you're at risk of type 2 diabetes. Potatoes break down quickly in your stomach, which creates a fast, steep rise in blood sugar.

In a 20-year Harvard study of 84,500 women, those who splurged on french fries just once a week raised their diabetes risk by 21 percent, compared with those who ate none. And five servings a week of any white potatoes, even baked ones, raised risk by 14 percent, compared with less than a half serving a week. Obese women were even more likely to get diabetes from eating a lot of potatoes.

Because this study found that instant, mashed, and baked spuds raise sugar the most, eat them only occasionally if you're trying to control blood sugar spikes. Avoid fries, too.

If you *do* indulge in that once-a-week spud, chill it first. Cool potatoes don't raise postmeal blood sugar levels as much as hot ones do, a 2004 study found. Researchers at the American University of Beirut had nine healthy men eat one of three test meals—hot boiled potatoes, cooled boiled potatoes, or white bread—on three separate mornings after fasting the night before. The researchers tested the volunteers' blood sugar, insulin, cholesterol, and triglyceride levels before and for 3 hours after each test meal.

The men's blood sugar levels were significantly higher 30 minutes after eating the hot potato, compared with the cooled one, and stayed high for 3 hours. And while the men's triglycerides dropped after they ate the cooled potatoes, levels increased after the hot spuds were eaten and stayed high for the 3-hour period.

WHAT IF I DON'T LIKE . . .
VEGETABLES?

Veggies are so key to the Diabetes Rescue Diet that there's no way to avoid them. However, there are a couple of ways to sneak them into your diet. The tips below won't give you all of the benefits of eating a wide variety of vegetables—you'll miss out on fiber, for example, which offers huge benefits for people with diabetes. But you'll get some of the benefits, which is better than none.

The most obvious alternative to eating veggies is to drink them. The most widely known brand of vegetable juice, V8, contains tomatoes, beets, carrots, celery, spinach, lettuce, parsley, and watercress. If you watch your salt intake, opt for the low-sodium version. You can also buy organic veggie juices at your local natural foods store.

Another option: Grate vegetables finely and add to other foods. To do this, buy a fine grater disk for your food processor. It'll mince those veggies into microscopic bits, which you can then hide in ground meat or spaghetti sauce. For the latter, try this: Grate 2 cups (total) of onions, garlic, carrots, beets, spinach, and zucchini, then sauté in olive oil. Add 4 cups of basic marinara sauce and simmer to an anonymous tomato flavor.

Or simply eat salsa. I recommend fresh salsa, which contains tomatoes, peppers, onions, and spices. You'll find it with the prechopped veggies in the produce section of your supermarket. Use it to top chicken, brown rice, or potatoes or even as an alternative to salad dressing.

A great way to enjoy your potato: Whip up a single serving of potato salad, made with chilled potatoes and prepared with vinaigrette. A 2005 Swedish study of 13 healthy people found that potato salad with olive oil and vinegar dressing raised blood sugar levels 43 percent less than a baked tater. The chilling and the vinegar increased the availability of a kind of fiber called resistant starch in the spuds, the study found. As the name suggests, resistant starch "resists" being digested. Because it doesn't enter your bloodstream, it stabilizes blood sugar levels and may lower diabetes risk. It can help avoid the blood sugar surge and insulin rise associated with eating potatoes.

Oh, and if you can, make your potato salad with new potatoes. They have the lowest amount of starch and thus the lowest glycemic index of any type of potato. New potatoes are not a separate variety of potato but immature versions of others that haven't grown enough to develop much starch. They're smaller than other types of potatoes. They also have thinner skins, so you don't even have to peel them.

Take Five and Thrive

Five servings of veggies a day—that's all it takes to reduce your risk of diabetes, avoid its complications, and protect your heart and arteries. "Servings" are counted in half cups and cups. One serving equals 1 cup of raw leafy vegetables; ½ cup of another vegetable, such as baby carrots or green beans; or 6 ounces of vegetable juice. So what does "five servings a day" look like? Here's a sample day.

Breakfast: bell peppers, broccoli, spinach, mushrooms, or tomatoes added to your egg or egg white omelet; or tomato or vegetable juice sipped with your meal (½ cup)

Midmorning snack: six baby carrots with hummus (½ cup)

Lunch: salad with romaine lettuce and other salad veggies (1½ cups)

Afternoon snack: leftover salad or veggies from last night's dinner or cut-up raw veggies (bell peppers, carrots, squash, broccoli) with dip (1 cup)

Dinner: 1 cup sautéed greens plus a serving of green beans or half a sweet potato (1½ cups)

Select your veggies not just for taste but with an eye for color—

greens, orange bell peppers and sweet potatoes, yellow squash, purple eggplant, red tomatoes, and white and red onions. The brighter a veggie's hue, the more antioxidant phytochemicals it contains, not to mention fiber, vitamins, and minerals.

Fresh veggies are expensive. But here's another surprise that will ease your mind (and wallet): Frozen produce is even more nutrient packed. That's because the moment produce is picked, it starts to lose nutrients, but freezing slows that loss.

A 2007 study found that the vitamin C content of fresh broccoli plummeted 56 percent in 7 days but dipped just 10 percent in a year's time when frozen at -4°F. In addition, the levels of disease-fighting antioxidants called anthocyanins and some minerals, including potassium (which helps control blood pressure), actually increased after freezing!

If you prefer vegetables fresh rather than frozen or canned, you'll definitely want to read the next section. It appears that, like most everything else, fresh veggies ain't what they used to be.

Punch Up Fresh Produce

I hate to burst the "fresh veggies are best" bubble, but consider this shocker: *The vegetables and fruits you buy in the produce aisle today aren't as nutritious as they were 30 years ago.* It's true—several studies have confirmed it.

In a 2004 study, researchers at the University of Texas, Austin, analyzed 43 fruits and vegetables from 1950 to 1999. They found reductions in vitamins, minerals, and protein. Using USDA data, they found that broccoli, for example, had 130 milligrams of calcium in 1950. Today, broccoli contains less than half that amount: 48 milligrams.

According to researchers who study this topic, it may be that the farming industry's desire to grow bigger vegetables faster results in this less-nutritious produce. The same things that speed growth—selective breeding and synthetic fertilizers—reduce fruits' and veggies' ability to synthesize nutrients or absorb them from the soil.

Organic produce is a different story. Because they don't use synthetic fertilizers, organic farmers put more stress on plants—and stressed-out plants protect themselves by producing phytochemicals. In a 10-year study, researchers at the University of California, Davis, found that organic tomatoes can have as many as 30 percent more phytochemicals than conventional ones. If you want to buy organic produce, you can—but you don't need to. The expert recommendations below can help put the nutrient punch back in your produce.

Go local. Unlike supermarket produce, which typically travels hundreds of miles before landing on store shelves, a farmers' market or pick-your-own place offers local, freshly harvested, in-season fare that's had a chance to ripen naturally—a process that amplifies the amount of phytonutrients.

Go bold. Look for the brightest veggies in the produce aisle. Typically, the brighter a vegetable's skin (a fruit's, too), the more phytochemicals it packs. One 2002 study found that darker-orange carrots contain more beta-carotene than the typical "orangey orange" carrots.

5-Minute Veggies, 5 Ways

- Stock up on frozen vegetables. You don't have to wash, peel, or chop. And you can nuke them! Remember, frozen veggies can actually be more nutritious.

- Buy premade supermarket salads. One of my favorites is the broccoli-cranberry slaw at Fresh Market—broccoli, carrots, red cabbage, dried cranberries, and sliced almonds dressed with oil and vinegar: healthy, delicious, and ready to eat when you pull off the top.

- The next time you grill burgers, toss on a skewer or two of veggies—cherry tomatoes; chunks of red, yellow, or orange bell peppers and onions; and thick slices of green and yellow squash.

- Toss thawed frozen or canned vegetables into pasta sauce.

- Pile your pizza with roasted vegetables, baked eggplant, mushrooms, onions, peppers, tomatoes, sun-dried tomatoes, broccoli, or spinach.

Go small. Pass up those huge FrankenVeggies. Plants can pass on only so many nutrients to the actual veggie (or fruit). If produce is smaller, its level of nutrients is typically more concentrated, research has found.

Cook gently. Some vegetables release more nutrients when they're cooked. For example, steamed broccoli and carrots are more nutritious than raw or boiled. (Gentle heat softens their cell walls, so your body can better access their nutrients.) And tomatoes release more of their primary phytochemical, lycopene, when you lightly sauté or roast them.

Use fast. The nutrients in most fruits and vegetables start to fade as soon as they're picked, so for optimal nutrition, eat all produce within a week of buying it.

10 Ways to Mediterraneanize Your Veggies

Okay, one way involves a wok. But most of the vegetable dishes below— from Greece, France, Italy, and Spain—will develop your appreciation for vegetables.

★ Instead of a plain old iceberg lettuce salad, treat yourself to a *horiatiki salata*—a Greek village salad. Combine sliced fresh tomatoes, green peppers, onions (red or white), and cucumbers. Toss in some Greek olives, capers, and crumbled feta cheese. Dress it with red wine vinegar and extra-virgin olive oil. Dust it with oregano. *Nostimos!* (Delicious!)

★ Italians love broccoli rabe, a variety of broccoli that's kin to both turnips and cabbage. Its taste is distinctive—its "bite" softens when it's sautéed in olive oil and garlic. To make it Italian style, rinse in cold water, shake, and remove the tough ends of the stalks. Some people like it as a cold salad: steamed, then cooled and dressed with oil, hot peppers, garlic, and other seasonings.

★ Grill vegetables—you'll develop a new appreciation for them, and it's simple. Cut any veggie into slices of consistent thickness and no more than ¾ to 1 inch. Soak vegetables in cold water for 30 minutes to keep them from drying out during grilling. Pat dry, then brush lightly with olive oil so they won't stick to the grill. Try tomatoes, mushrooms, bell peppers (red, yellow, or orange), and onions. You can even grill asparagus!

★ I like roasted veggies, too, especially in the winter. Sweet carrots and red onion, tender baby Brussels sprouts, or mellow squash drizzled with tart vinegar—the combination delivers a new burst of flavor in every bite.

★ In the Catalan region of northern Spain, sautéed Swiss chard with raisins and pine nuts is an everyday side dish. (Or use spinach, if you prefer—the Catalans do.) In a large saucepan, bring 2 cups water to a boil. Add 1 teaspoon salt and 2 cups coarsely chopped Swiss chard (remove the stems first) or spinach. Cover and cook until tender, maybe 15 minutes. Drain the greens in a colander and set aside. Heat ¼ cup olive oil over high heat in a skillet. Add ¼ cup pine nuts (available in most large supermarkets), stir, then add the Swiss chard or spinach and ¼ cup raisins and mix well. Stir until all the ingredients are heated through, then serve.

★ Pair pasta with two greens—say, broccoli or broccoli rabe and zucchini. Top with feta and Parmesan.

★ Stuff orange, red, or yellow bell peppers with a mixture of brown rice and beans, toss 'em in the slow cooker, and cover with tomato sauce. The sauce will keep them moist as they cook.

★ Use leftover veggies like red peppers and broccoli to prepare an oven-fresh homemade pizza. I like mine topped with creamy goat cheese.

★ The French summer vegetable stew ratatouille—made with chunks of tomato, onion, eggplant, and zucchini—is as delicious as it is versatile. Use it as a filling for omelets with a little feta or goat cheese, or toss with cooked pasta and grated Parmesan. It also makes a wonderful chunky topping for grilled or baked fish.

★ Break out your wok and stir-fry a sizzling selection of broccoli, red peppers, cabbage, and snow peas. Add fresh grated ginger and hot chile peppers for heat.

Rescuer No. 6

BEANS

⅓ to ½ cup each day

I eat beans like a Mediterranean—they hit my plate or bowl almost every day. My default lunch is hummus, the savory dip made with chickpeas, lemon, parsley, and spices. My wife's bean, vegetable, and greens soup packs half the Diabetes Rescue Diet in one bowl. Black beans and chickpeas top my salads.

Technically, beans (like black beans, pintos, and kidney beans) and peas (like split peas and lentils) are the mature form of legumes—plants whose seeds come in pods with two halves. (In fact, a peanut isn't a nut at all; it's a legume!) But to keep things simple, I call 'em all beans. Whatever you call them, they're delicious, cheap, and easy to make.

And if you want to live forever (or at least a long time), eat beans. A

Beans Up, Belly Fat Down

Want to take a little off the middle? Bean up! People who eat ¾ cup of beans a day have smaller waist sizes than those who skip beans in favor of other proteins, a 2008 study in the *Journal of the American College of Nutrition* found. They have lower blood pressure, too.

Even if you eat a modified Mediterranean diet that includes beans, you'll pack less belly fat, a study of 497,308 men and women in 10 European countries suggests.

Researchers in health centers throughout Europe wanted to study the link between body fat and a diet that included, but wasn't limited to, components of a traditional Mediterranean diet. They scored the participants' diets based on nine nutritional factors, some of which—like bean consumption—are part of a Mediterranean diet. But the researchers also included foods that Europeans typically eat a lot of, but Mediterranean people eat in smaller amounts, like meat and dairy. This "European style" Mediterranean diet was linked to a lower waist circumference, the study found. So even doing modified Mediterranean may slim your belly, the researchers said.

study of people over the age of 70 in four countries around the globe found that bean consumption was the strongest predictor of longer life. Just 20 grams a day make a big difference in lowering risk of death. That's less than two-thirds of an ounce. Eating, say, 3 or 4 ounces a day reduces mortality risk by around 25 percent.

Beans are especially healthy for people with diabetes. Their hefty amounts of fiber slow the release of glucose into your bloodstream, dramatically smoothing out blood sugar spikes that often occur after meals. If you have diabetes, that matters a lot—such postmeal blood sugar surges can raise the risk of heart disease, research has found. In one 2006 study of 529 men and women with type 2 diabetes, high after-meal peaks raised the risk of cardiovascular events like heart attack by five times! In men, the risk doubled. The after-lunch blood sugar rise was especially dangerous. (Moral: Eat beans with lunch!)

Beans are also an excellent source of protein, and unlike red meat, they're low in saturated fat, the kind that plugs up arteries and can lead to heart disease.

As it does with dairy, the Diabetes Rescue Diet includes more beans than the latest Dietary Guidelines suggest, but I bet you'll be surprised at just how small that amount really is. (I'm not talking a hill of beans!) So if you're not eating beans now, prepare to spoon them up. Dry or canned, in whatever variety you like, they'll help you manage your diabetes, protect your heart, and shrink your belly.

"Full of Beans" Beats Diabetes

The complications of uncontrolled blood sugar aren't pleasant to consider. Vision loss. Kidney failure. You know the rest. But here's the good news: Keep your HbA1c in target range, evidence suggests, and risk of these complications—which also include heart disease and stroke—goes down.

HbA1c is short for *hemoglobin A1c*. It's a component of hemoglobin, the oxygen-carrying pigment that gives blood its red color. Glucose in the blood attaches to HbA1c. So the higher the glucose concentration in blood, the higher the level of HbA1c.

That's why your doctor tests your HbA1c every 2 to 3 months. Daily glucose tests are snapshots, but the HbA1c test gives you the big picture of how you're managing your diabetes overall.

The A1c goal for most people with diabetes is below 7 percent. A growing body of research suggests that the best way to achieve this goal is to reduce postmeal blood sugar surges. And what you eat at those meals can help or hurt.

That's where beans enter the picture. Because they're packed with fiber, beans are digested slowly, resulting in a gradual, gentle rise in blood sugar. German researchers showed this when they fed nine people with type 2 diabetes a small amount of two different carbohydrate foods: dried peas or potatoes. After the participants ate 1.2 ounces of dried peas, their postmeal rise in blood sugar was one-third of what it was after they ate an equal amount of spuds.

There's more. In a small Canadian study, a breakfast of lentils reduced glucose rise by a huge 71 percent, compared with bread. Not only that, but those morning lentils flattened the blood sugar rise produced by lunch, 4 hours later, by a stunning 38 percent.

But can a bean-rich diet lower the risk of type 2 diabetes itself?

Meet Your Beans

Y ou think you know beans, and maybe you are familiar with the more common varieties. But I'm betting that there are more than a few on this list that you've never tried. Since you're eating like an Italian or Greek now, seek them out (perhaps in natural foods stores) and give them a try.

Black adzuki beans: While they look a lot like common black beans, black adzukis have a sweet flavor and are relatively easy to digest, so they won't make you as gassy as other types of beans. They also don't take as long to cook.

Black beans: Sometimes called turtle beans, these small oval beans with an ebony skin have a mild, sweet, earthy taste and soft texture. They're a staple of Latin American and Caribbean cuisine and are used to make side dishes, soups, dips, and salads.

Black-eyed peas: Also known as cowpeas, these white beans are marked by a small black "eye" and have a creamy texture and distinctive flavor. They cook rapidly—no presoaking needed.

Cannellini beans: You've probably eaten these Italian beans in minestrone soup or a bean salad. White, medium size, and flat, they're known for their smooth texture and nutty flavor.

Chickpeas (garbanzos): These beige-to-pale-yellow round beans have a nutlike taste. They're especially popular in many Middle Eastern and Indian dishes such as hummus, falafel, and curry.

Cranberry beans: These small round beans, known for their creamy texture, have a subtle, nutlike flavor. They're pretty, too—ivory, with red markings that disappear when they're cooked. They're commonly used in Italian soups and stews.

Several studies suggest it can. In 2008, researchers from the Vanderbilt University Cancer Institute and the Shanghai Cancer Institute analyzed food questionnaires filled out by 64,227 middle-aged Chinese women with no history of diabetes or cardiovascular disease, who were followed for more than 4 years.

Fava beans: These large tan beans have a strong flavor and have been around for ages, and they work well in side dishes, soups, or salads.

Great Northern beans: These flat, medium-size, white beans take on the flavors of the foods with which they are cooked. That's why the French use them to make cassoulet, a white bean casserole, and why they're used in this country to make Boston baked beans.

Lima beans: There are two types—baby, which have a rich, buttery flavor; and large, sometimes called butter beans, which also have a mild flavor. Both are excellent in soups, stews, and casseroles.

Navy beans: Also known as pea beans, these small, white, oval beans have a mild flavor and powdery texture. They're typically used in baked beans, soups, and stews.

Pink beans: These beans are much like pintos (below) but smaller and rounder. They're often used to make chili and refried beans.

Pinto beans: When cooked, this oval bean's mottled beige-and-brown skin turns brown. Their earthy flavor makes pintos perfect for Tex-Mex and Mexican bean dishes, including refried beans.

Red beans: These are similar to red kidney beans, only smaller, rounder, and darker. In the Southwest, they're often used in refried beans and chili. In Louisiana, they're used to make the classic red beans and rice.

Rice beans: Yes, they look like rice, but unlike rice, they cook in 15 minutes—and you don't have to soak them. Some people use them instead of rice to make risotto.

MAXIMIZERS

Beans

There's really no "healthiest bean." Thank goodness—with so many varieties and flavors to choose from, it would be terrible to have to eat just one or two types to get their health benefits. You can cook using either canned or dried beans. I recommend dried beans when possible because they are often a little less expensive, easier to store, and don't come in BPA-lined aluminum cans, reducing your exposure to the potentially hazardous hormone-mimicking plastic. Dried beans may not look as appetizing at first as their canned counterparts, but there are definitely ways to pump up their flavor and tenderness.

First, start with fresh dried beans—that is, beans under a year old. If they've languished in your pantry for more than a year, they may not get tender when you cook them, no matter how long they're in the pot or slow cooker.

If you have hard water, your cooked beans might be a little on the tough side. This old trick will soften them right up: Add ¼ teaspoon baking soda for each pound of beans. Use a bit less if your beans are fresh. Although you're cooking in hard water, too much baking soda might actually make fresh beans mushy.

Timing is important, too. Add salt and acidic foods, such as tomatoes, vinegar, and lemon (molasses, too), near the end of the cooking time, so these ingredients don't toughen the beans' skins.

The results were spectacular. Women who ate the most legumes of any type—⅓ cup, on average—slashed their diabetes risk by a whopping 38 percent! Those who ate the most soybeans (about ¼ cup) lowered their risk even more—by 47 percent. (Eating lots of other soy products, however, didn't lower risk.) That's a lot of protection from a little hill of beans.

In 2009, researchers from Canada examined the results of 41 clinical trials, which involved 1,674 people, on the effects of beans and peas on blood sugar control. Eleven trials looked at beans and peas alone, with the experimental "dose" averaging about ½ cup a day, and found that a high legume intake alone lowered both fasting blood glucose by 80 percent and insulin levels by 50 percent. In 19 studies, beans given as part of a high-fiber or low-glycemic-index diet improved HbA1c by 0.5 percent, on average. That's as good as or better than some diabetes medications!

Give a Toot for Your Heart

Everyone knows the funny ditty about beans being good for your heart, but that's not just song and dance. There's compelling evidence that beans really do protect your heart and arteries.

In one of the latest studies, from 2011, researchers at Tulane University in New Orleans analyzed data from 10 clinical trials that looked at the effect of legume consumption on cholesterol. After the numbers were crunched, the evidence was clear: Beans clobbered both total and LDL cholesterol. Specifically, of the 268 people (mostly middle-aged men) included in the studies, the total cholesterol of the biggest bean eaters was 12 points lower, on average, than those who ate the fewest beans—and their LDL cholesterol levels were 8 points lower. The researchers called out beans' soluble fiber and their plant nutrients, such as phytosterols, for contributing to the cholesterol-lowering effects.

This study is important because previous research focused mainly on the cholesterol-lowering effects of the soybean. Now, soybeans are a fine bean, but they're less commonly eaten, at least in America. So this study proved that beans and peas can be cholesterol busters, too.

Some studies have even looked at specific types of beans. For example, pinto beans, which are typically used in many dishes like chili, baked beans, and Mexican foods, hammer down bad cholesterol, a 2007 study conducted at Arizona State University found. Just a half cup a day lowered total cholesterol, including LDL, by up to 8 percent. In this study, the key to pintos' heart healthiness was its abundance of fiber, long known to slow the rate and amount of absorption of cholesterol in certain foods.

The humble bean may also help protect against heart attack. In a 2005 Costa Rican study, researchers studied 2,119 survivors of a sudden heart attack and 2,119 people with no history of a heart attack. They found that 69 percent of these folks ate at least one serving (⅓ cup) of cooked beans per day. The biggest bean eaters cut their risk of heart attack by a staggering 38 percent, compared with those who never ate beans or had them less than once a month.

The more beans/fewer heart attacks association didn't surprise the team. The researchers noted beans' nutritional bounty: magnesium,

WHAT IF I DON'T LIKE . . .
BEANS?

Then give peas a chance. Seriously. I don't mean green peas, which is technically a starchy veggie, but dried peas, which include cowpeas (also known as black-eyed peas), green split peas, and yellow split peas.

Split pea soup is a good option for nonbeanies. Its texture is smooth, and its flavor mild. This easy recipe for split pea soup is perfect for lunch or a light dinner and—like the peas themselves—is low in fat and filled with nutrients and fiber. It makes four servings, so you'll have enough for leftovers (and leftover pea soup is the best!).

Set a pot over medium-high heat for 1 minute. Add ⅓ tablespoon olive oil and swirl to coat the bottom. Heat for 30 seconds. Add ¼ cup each chopped celery and onion, ¼ teaspoon dried thyme, and 1 bay leaf and stir. Cook, stirring occasionally, for 4 minutes, or until softened. Add ½ pound green split peas and 4 cups chicken or vegetable broth and bring almost to a boil. Reduce the heat to medium-low. Cover partially and simmer for about 2 hours, or until the peas are very soft. Remove the bay leaf and discard. In the bowl of a food processor fitted with a metal blade, in a blender, or with an immersion blender, puree the mixture until smooth. Add ¼ teaspoon salt and ½ teaspoon hot-pepper sauce. If the mixture is too thick, add water, if desired.

copper, fiber, and alpha-linolenic acid, all of which have been found to improve insulin sensitivity, normalize cholesterol levels, reduce the tendency of blood to clot, and reduce the cell-damaging process of oxidation. And, of course, beans' complex carbohydrates lower glycemic load.

Don't think you have to cook beans, either: Just 6.5 ounces a day of beans in tomato sauce, right out of the can, lowered cholesterol by more than 10 percent in 3 weeks, a University of Kentucky study found.

Maximum Power, Minimum Gas

The most recent Dietary Guidelines actually reduced the recommended weekly amount of beans from 3 cups to 1½ cups. The Diabetes Rescue Diet, however, recommends the amount shown in studies to lower blood sugar and protect the heart—from ⅓ to ½ cup a day.

Once you start to eat beans every day, you'll be amazed at what you can tuck them into. (I'll give you some different yet easy suggestions later on.) It doesn't matter whether you use dried or canned—both are nutritious. Some beans and peas, like lentils, cook in a few hours, and you can always toss them in your slow cooker overnight.

If you have time to soak dried beans, go for it—they tend to be cheaper. If you're pressed for time, boil the beans for 2 minutes, then cover the pot and soak for 1 to 4 hours. When you're ready to cook the beans, discard the soaking water, cover the beans with fresh water, and add 2 tablespoons of oil, which will keep them from foaming as they cook.

If you're in no hurry, cover the beans with water and soak them overnight (12 hours or longer). Then cover them with fresh water, add the oil, and cook. Store your dried beans in an airtight container in a cool, dry place, like your pantry. They'll keep for up to 1 year.

If you're a lazy or harried cook, like me, use canned beans. Keep a few different types in your pantry, so you'll always have the makings for a quick meal. Just drain them in a colander and rinse under cold water to get rid of the extra sodium.

Of course, the downside of eating beans is gas, especially if you haven't been eating them regularly. The tooting happens because beans contain complex sugars that require special enzymes to break them down. If you don't have these enzymes in your digestive tract, the sugars ferment, and you toot.

If you use dry beans, changing the water from time to time during soaking will reduce those gas-causing sugars. It also helps to cook them until you can mash them easily with a fork—and you can change the water while you're cooking them, too. Or simply buy a gas-reducing enzyme tablet (such as Beano) at the supermarket or drugstore. Take it just before you take your first bite of beans. Problem solved.

9 Ways to Bean Up Your Day

There are three simple ways to get beans into your diet—add them to salads, soups, and pasta sauces. But if you're looking to go beyond those tried-and-true tips, these suggestions are almost as quick and easy.

★ Scrambling eggs for breakfast? Add some south-of-the-border zing with ¼ cup black beans and salsa to taste.

★ The next time you make homemade pizza, top it with a cup of your favorite beans just before you add the cheese. Think of them as the healthy alternative to sausage or pepperoni. Black beans are perfect—they're small and have a mild flavor.

★ As much as I love my chickpea hummus, you can make it with many other beans, including lentils and black beans. Simply whir the beans in your food processor; add seasonings and spices, a squirt of lemon juice, and a drizzle of olive oil; blend; and serve.

★ Whip up a taco salad Diabetes Rescue style. Add ½ cup rinsed, drained canned black beans to 2 cups baby greens. Top with ¼ cup salsa, sprinkle with feta or reduced-fat shredded Cheddar cheese, and garnish with 2 tablespoons chopped avocado.

★ I often eat lentil soup for breakfast (yes, breakfast) or lunch, especially on cold, wet days. Another way to get your lentils: Whip up some dal, the Indian dish of split peas or lentils cooked with onions and spices. Here's just one of many dal recipes: Wash 1½ cups red or brown lentils or yellow or green split peas in cold water. In a medium pot, cover the peas or lentils with 4 cups water. Add 2 whole dried chiles, ¼ teaspoon turmeric, and ½ teaspoon salt. Bring to a boil, reduce the heat, and simmer, stirring often, until very tender (about 30 minutes for lentils and 45 minutes for peas). If necessary, add more water, ½ cup at a time, to prevent sticking.

Meanwhile, heat 2 tablespoons olive oil in a small pan. Add ½ teaspoon cumin seeds and sauté for 10 to 15 seconds.

Mex Meal Secrets

Jack and Jane, who both have type 2 diabetes, go into a Mexican restaurant. They order the same meal: a bean-and-cheese burrito on a flour tortilla. Both burritos contain equal amounts of carbs, fat, and calories. But after the meal, Jane's blood sugar rises significantly less than Jack's. What's her secret?

Simple: Jane ordered a tortilla made with whole rather than refried beans.

The "secret" seems to lie in the cells of the beans themselves, according to a study conducted at the Stanford University School of Medicine. For two mornings in a row, the researchers gave nine people with type 2 diabetes a meal containing beans. These beans were processed by methods that left their cell walls either damaged or undamaged—smooshed or unsmooshed, if you will. The meal: a bean-and-cheese burrito on a flour tortilla.

When the volunteers ate the tortilla made with the unsmooshed beans, their blood sugar was 171 mg/dL, compared with 212 mg/dL when they ate the tortilla with the smooshed beans. Beans with intact cell walls seem to help blood sugar rise more slowly and gradually than those with damaged cell walls, the researchers said.

The lesson here: Next time you dine at a Mexican restaurant, ask the waiter to have the cook put whole beans, not *frijoles refritos,* in your tortilla. Most Mexican places offer whole beans—they just don't put them in tortillas because they tend to tumble out, while refried beans stay put. But so what? Your blood sugar will thank you.

Add 1 cup chopped onions and 1 teaspoon grated fresh ginger and sauté for 5 to 10 minutes, or until the onions begin to brown. When the lentils are tender, discard the peppers. Stir in the onions and 1 tablespoon lemon juice, and salt to taste.

★ Have a bean burrito for lunch—it takes about 2 minutes to make. Microwave a whole grain tortilla until warm and soft, and transfer to a plate. Spread ½ cup fat-free refried beans—or ½ cup cooked whole pinto beans—down the center of the tortilla. Top with your choice of shredded lettuce, diced tomato or onion, and 1 tablespoon guacamole. Add a shot of salsa. Fold the bottom end of the tortilla toward the center, then roll it around the filling.

★ Spoon cooked lentils (maybe some leftover dal) on half a whole grain bagel or a piece of sourdough or pumpernickel toast.

★ For a quick, tasty snack, spoon 2 tablespoons garbanzo beans into each of 4 large romaine lettuce leaves. Top each with a few strips of jarred roasted red pepper, and garnish with chopped onions and pine nuts.

★ Whip up a cold bean salad using canned black beans, fresh or frozen corn kernels, and chopped onion and tomato. To intensify the flavor, splurge on chopped mint or cilantro. Dress the salad with olive oil and a dash of balsamic vinegar.

Rescuer No. **7**

FRUITS

Three to four servings a day

Yes, people with diabetes can eat fruit: everyday favorites like crisp apples, juicy berries, and creamy bananas; exotic fruits like papaya, mango, and bright-green kiwifruit. I eat yogurt-topped fresh fruit for breakfast every morning, and so can you.

In fact, if you have diabetes or are at risk of it, you *should* eat fruit. Like veggies, fruits are packed with fiber, vitamins, minerals, and plant compounds with powerful antioxidant properties. These compounds, called phytochemicals, protect against diabetes, cardiovascular disease, and cancer, research suggests. You can thank phytochemicals for the crayon-bright hues of berries, watermelon, citrus fruits, and blue-black plums and grapes.

As a great source of vitamin C, fruit also helps prevent the damage that high blood sugar wreaks on cells and arteries. As a bonus, fruit eaters tend to be slimmer: Women at a healthy weight eat one more serving of fruit and get more fiber and less fat per day than those who are overweight, a study published in the *Journal of the American Dietetic Association* found. What's more, because fruit is low in fat and sodium, it's easy on your blood pressure and cholesterol—always good news if you have diabetes.

Fruit contains a lot of good stuff—and it contains carbohydrates, too. So if you have diabetes, count fruit as part of your meal plan, and keep track of serving sizes (this chapter will help with that). Some fruits do contain more sugar than others, but the amount of carbohydrates in a serving of fruit affects blood sugar more than the source of those carbohydrates, whether they're starch or sugar. It's time to let the "people with diabetes can't eat fruit" myth fade away and enjoy the natural sweetness—and health benefits.

Solid Science, Sweet Protection

Want to slash your risk of diabetes by 28 percent? I have three words for you: *Eat an apple.* In a study of 38,018 women, those who ate at least one apple a day were 28 percent less likely to develop diabetes than those who didn't, researchers at Brigham and Women's Hospital and Harvard Medical School found. (Eat the skin, too—see "Meet the Maximizers: Apple Skins" on page 104.)

This study didn't directly link specific plant chemicals in apples to the reduction in diabetes risk. But apples are rich in polyphenols, as are tea, berries, and wine. Scientists have been studying polyphenols for more than a decade, and they're making new discoveries. For example, polyphenols may benefit blood sugar, a 2010 review article conducted at the University of Eastern Finland suggests. There are two types of polyphenols—nonflavonoids and flavonoids. One of the most-studied flavonoids is quercetin, and apples are brimming with it.

Foods or drinks rich in polyphenols have been shown in more than 70 test-tube and animal studies to reduce blood sugar levels after meals and improve the action of insulin, the review noted. Polyphenols might offer these benefits in several ways. The flavonoids in

Fresh, Frozen, or Canned?

I don't care whether you eat fresh, frozen, or canned fruits, as long as you eat them. Which one you choose depends on your preferences and budget.

Fresh: If you prefer fresh fruits, that's great. Just know that once they're harvested, heat, light, and time break down some of their nutrients. So the amount of nutrients in your fruit bowl depends on how long ago those fruits were picked, how many days they spent in transit to your supermarket, and how long they sat before you ate them. For the greatest nutritional value and flavor, buy fruit in season from your local farmers' market or a roadside stand.

If you opt for fresh fruit, make sure there are no bruises or spots. It should smell fresh and be ripe enough to eat either now or in a few days. And no matter which variety you buy, wash fruit before you eat it. There's no need to buy special washes. Simply rub it briskly under running water to remove dirt and surface microorganisms.

Frozen: If cost and convenience are your top concerns, it's fine to opt for frozen (or canned) fruits, which are generally processed immediately upon harvest, when their nutrient content is at its peak. The variety is very good, especially in frozen fruits. For example, it's a good bet that you'll find mango and papaya chunks in the frozen-foods aisle.

Canned: Opt for fruits packed in their own juice, rather than light or heavy syrups.

apples may inhibit digestive enzymes (alpha-amylase and alpha-glucosidase) that help break down carbohydrates into glucose, so carbs are converted to glucose more slowly. Other polyphenols might also reduce the absorption of glucose from the digestive tract, stimulate the beta cells of the pancreas to secrete insulin, or activate insulin receptors, which helps glucose get into cells where it's needed.

But it's not just apples that benefit blood sugar, a study of more than 70,000 women found. Researchers at the Tulane University School of Public Health in New Orleans looked into the link between intake of fruit, vegetables, and fruit juice and the development of diabetes. Using dietary data from the landmark Nurses' Health Studies, the researchers divided 71,346 female nurses into five groups based on their consumption of these foods. In 18 years, 4,529 of the nurses developed diabetes.

The nurses who ate three servings of whole fruit a day had an 18 percent lower risk of diabetes, the study found. But one additional daily serving of fruit juice raised risk by the same amount—18 percent. (For the record, a single additional serving of green leafy vegetables was associated with a 9 percent reduction in diabetes risk.)

Fruit juice is loaded with sugar, and the body quickly absorbs this liquid sugar, the study noted. The bottom line: Think twice about swapping sugar-laden drinks like soda for fruit juice in a bid to choose a healthier drink.

Fruit Is Heart-Smart, Too

Taking care of your heart is a top priority if you have diabetes. Several landmark studies clearly show that fruit is an essential part of a heart-healthy diet.

For example, in a 2003 study, researchers led by Demosthenes B. Panagiotakos, MD, looked at the link between coronary heart disease risk and fruit and vegetable intake in 1,878 Greek men and women—800 with heart disease and 1,078 healthy people. With the help of food questionnaires, the researchers assessed these peoples' diets, including their fruit and vegetable intake, for roughly 2 years.

The more fruits and veggies they ate, the more health benefits they reaped, the study showed. After the researchers adjusted for smoking, high blood pressure and cholesterol, and other standard cardiovascular risk factors, they found that people who ate five or more fruits a day slashed their risk of coronary heart disease a staggering 72 percent, compared with those who ate less than one serving a day. Even consuming vegetables more than 3 days a week was associated with a 70 percent lower risk, compared with those who ate none at all. And get this: *For every one piece of fruit consumed per day, there was a 10 percent reduction in coronary risk.*

I'm not advising that you eat five pieces of fruit a day, but in this study, the association between fruit and heart health is clear.

In another 2003 study conducted in Japan and published in the medical journal *Stroke*, researchers collected data on 40,349 Japanese men and women. The researchers wanted to study the protective effect of a diet rich in fruits and vegetables on total stroke mortality and stroke's two main subtypes—ischemic stroke, caused by a clot in a blood vessel that supplies blood to the brain, and hemorrhagic stroke, which occurs when a weakened blood vessel ruptures. During the 18-year study period, 1,926 people died of stroke.

People who ate fruits and green-yellow vegetables every day were 20 to 40 percent less likely to suffer a fatal stroke than those who ate these whole foods less than once a week, the study found. Also, eating fruit every day was associated with a 35 percent reduction in risk of total stroke in men and a 25 percent risk reduction in women. These reductions were equally strong for both ischemic and hemorrhagic strokes. The vitamins, nutrients, and phytochemicals in fruits and veggies are most likely the reason for the reduced risk, the study said—many have been found to lower and control high blood pressure, a major risk factor for stroke.

Vitamin C: Fruity-licious Diabetes Protection

Do you want to lower your diabetes risk by two-thirds? Then belly up to berries, say yes to citrus, and treat your tastebuds to cantaloupe and kiwifruit.

In a 2008 study of 21,831 healthy people, the top 20 percent with the highest blood levels of vitamin C—suggestive of a high fruit and veggie intake—had a 62 percent lower risk of diabetes, compared with those in the lowest fifth, researchers at Addenbrooke's Hospital and the University of Cambridge in England found. Fruit and vegetable intake was also protective; those whose intake was in the top fifth slashed their diabetes risk by 22 percent, compared with those with the lowest intake. The vitamin may prevent the buildup of free radicals, which damage cells in a way that interferes with glucose metabolism and can cause diabetes.

Women with the highest blood levels of C ate an average of 6.5 servings of fruits and veggies per day, so if you have diabetes or are at

Apples Peel Down Cholesterol and More!

In 2004, a group at Cornell University looked at a very large number of studies about fruit and vegetable consumption and how it related to disease protection. They concluded that apples "were most consistently related" to reduced risk of type 2 diabetes, heart disease, and cancer, compared with other fruits and vegetables.

As this book was being written, a new study came out showing that apples may be even healthier than has been widely believed. Researchers at Florida State University had 160 postmenopausal women eat a small amount of either dried prunes or dried apples every day for a year. Researcher Bahram Arjmandi, PhD, RD, reported that "incredible changes in the apple-eating women happened by 6 months—they experienced a 23 percent decrease in LDL cholesterol"—known as the "bad" cholesterol.

Dr. Arjmandi said he never expected such a dramatic drop, which was accompanied by a 4 percent rise in HDL ("good") cholesterol. In addition, signs of inflammation of the arteries were reduced.

He added that though the daily snack of dried apples contained about 240 calories, the women didn't gain weight. In fact, they lost an average of 3.3 pounds.

If you want to follow this plan, the daily amount of dried apples was about 2½ ounces. The good thing about dried apples as opposed to fresh is that you can carry them easily in your belt pack or purse and eat some whenever you want a snack.

risk of it, enjoy the high-C fruits below. (Don't skimp on C-rich veggies like broccoli, red bell peppers, and kale, though.)

★ Kiwifruit (70 milligrams per fruit)

★ Orange (70 milligrams per fruit)

★ Strawberries (49 milligrams per ½ cup)

★ Cantaloupe (47 milligrams per ¼ medium melon)

★ Papaya (43 milligrams per ½ cup)

★ Grapefruit, white and red (39 milligrams per ½ grapefruit)

★ Raspberries (16 milligrams per ½ cup)

★ Blueberries (7 milligrams per ½ cup)

★ Peach (6.5 milligrams per fruit)

★ Apple (6 milligrams per fruit)

If you're a postmenopausal woman with diabetes, here's another good reason to reach for high-C fruits: It may be better for your cardiovascular health than popping large doses of vitamin C supplements.

In a 2004 study, researchers led by the University of Minnesota's School of Public Health followed 1,923 postmenopausal women already diagnosed with diabetes, 513 of whom died of cardiovascular disease in the 15 years the researchers followed them. Those who took 300 milligrams or more of vitamin C a day in supplement form were twice as likely to die of heart disease or stroke as those who didn't, the study found.

It may be that the vitamin C in food is "balanced biochemically," the researchers said, while high doses of just one antioxidant may disturb the body's balance of antioxidants and pro-oxidants (chemicals that speed cell damage by creating oxidative stress). Another key finding: High intakes of C from food didn't increase the risk of cardiovascular-related death.

Berries: Nature's Candy

I love all kinds of berries, and their health benefits are as sweet as their taste. A Tufts University study found that berries contain more anthocyanins—ultrapowerful antioxidants and the pigments that make blueberries blue, strawberries red, and blackberries black—than any other fruit. And the darker the berry, the greater the antioxidant protection, researchers say.

Berries are especially good for your ticker. Research suggests that their antioxidant power helps reduce the buildup of "bad" LDL cholesterol that can lead to heart disease and stroke. In a 2008 Finnish study of 72 people with heart disease risk factors, those who ate berries for 8 weeks had a 7 percent drop in blood pressure and a 5 percent boost in "good" HDL cholesterol. Let's take a look at the four most popular berries.

Blueberries: In a 2010 study of 32 obese, insulin-resistant people, researchers at Louisiana State University randomly assigned 15 participants to drink a smoothie made with 22.5 grams of freeze-dried blueberry powder (roughly equivalent to 1 cup of whole blueberries) twice a day; the other 17 drank a blueberry-free placebo smoothie. After 6 weeks, 67 percent of the blueberry group experienced a 10 percent or greater improvement in insulin sensitivity, compared with 41 percent of people in the placebo group. Although this study used freeze-dried blueberry powder, the research team conducted a study

---

MEET THE MAXIMIZERS

Apple Skins

I'm not one to peel my apples—too much fuss, and I actually like the texture and taste. I also like that eating the skin delivers every last bit of diabetes protection that apples have to offer.

While apple flesh contains phytochemicals, the skins are a concentrated source. That's because these compounds defend apples from dangers like birds, bugs, and environmental stress. Eat the skins and you reap those protective benefits.

In a Canadian study, researchers tested antioxidant levels in eight different varieties of apples. Red Delicious came out on top. In fact, the skin of a Red Delicious contains six times the antioxidants as in the flesh, the study found. The skins of Cortland, Golden Delicious, and McIntosh apples, among other varieties tested, contained fewer antioxidants. But in every variety tested, the skin packed significantly more antioxidants than the apple itself.

That was a test on apples, though. Another one, on people, shows

---

before this one that used whole blueberries and found that they reduced blood-sugar levels.

Raspberries: One cup nets you a hefty 8 grams of fiber for just 64 calories. Plus, these soft, red, melt-on-your-tongue berries have almost 50 percent more antioxidant activity than strawberries and three times that of kiwis, according to a 2005 Dutch study published in the journal *BioFactors*. Vitamin C accounts for about 20 percent of raspberries' total antioxidant capacity, and anthocyanins account for 25 percent, the researchers said. But more than 50 percent of that antioxidant punch comes from ellagitannins. These phytochemicals usually occur in leaves and bark, but in the raspberry, they also end up in the fruit.

compelling evidence of this fruit's power to thwart diabetes. In a Finnish study of 10,000 people, those who ate the most apples and other foods high in the phytochemical quercetin slashed their risk of death from diabetes and heart disease by 20 percent.

Eating unpeeled apples may even fight the early stages of diabetes, a 2010 study found. Researchers at the University of Massachusetts in Amherst evaluated 10 types of apples for their potential to manage diabetes. They found that, compared with other varieties, Honeycrisp and Red Delicious apples contain 10 to 15 percent more soluble phenolics, a group of natural compounds with powerful antioxidant properties. Just one apple can provide up to 50 milligrams of total soluble phenolics, with 25 percent of that coming from the peel alone, the study said.

I was happy to hear that Honeycrisp apples are top ranked—they've been my favorite apple for years now. But you can eat whatever variety you like, as long as you eat the skin, the study says.

If you must peel your apples, consider Northern Spy or Cortland. In the Canadian study, both of those varieties had more antioxidants in the flesh than Red Delicious did.

WHAT IF I DON'T LIKE . . .

PEELING, SKINNING, OR CHOPPING FRESH FRUIT?

Do what I do—choose no-fuss fruits. While I love kiwifruit, mangoes, and melons, I am fairly lazy when it comes to food prep, so I tend to favor berries, grapes, apples, and pears. No slicing, no dicing. I just wash and enjoy.

You can also let someone do the work for you. These days, you can pick up prewashed, cut-up fresh fruit at almost any supermarket and even most convenience stores. Another option: Buy frozen or canned fruit. Thaw one serving of mango or berries, or open a can of fruit packed in its own juice, and you're done.

Strawberries: Strawberries are a great source of fiber, packing 4 grams in one serving (1¼ cups). They also contain more vitamin C than any other berry; just one serving nets you 176 percent of the Daily Value. Their antioxidants, which include ellagic acid and anthocyanins, may help prevent the oxidation of LDL cholesterol.

Blackberries: These beauties are loaded with fiber; ¾ cup supplies 6 grams. And like black Mission figs, purple grapes, and black/purple plums, blackberries are loaded with anthocyanins, too.

Focus on 15

If you have diabetes, aim for three to four servings of fruit a day. To keep your blood sugar steady, all you need to do is pay attention to serving size.

If you have diabetes, one serving of fruit should contain 15 grams of carbohydrates. The size of the serving depends on the fruit's carbohydrate content. Although you can eat a larger portion of a low-carbohydrate fruit, the key is to keep one serving to 15 grams of carbs. Whether you eat a low-carb or high-carb type, the effect on your blood sugar is the same.

To reduce any sugar spike, eat fruit with a meal or as dessert. And be aware that when it comes to fruit, one whole fruit may be more than one serving. I don't know what you see in the produce aisle, but I see many fruits that are huge—for example, two or three apples might weigh a pound or more! In that case, count half of the apple as one serving and wrap up the other half for later.

By the way, fruit juice and dried fruit are so concentrated in sugar that 15 grams of carbs of either one is a pretty small amount. For example, a serving of fruit juice ranges from ⅓ cup to ½ cup, and one serving of dried fruit is just 2 tablespoons. This doesn't mean you can't have fruit juice in the morning or raisins in your oatmeal, but it does mean you can't have much of either.

The cheat sheet below gives you serving sizes of many common fruits. All portions are considered one serving and, except where indicated, contain 15 grams of carbohydrates or less per serving. Those with an asterisk (*) are considered low- or medium-GI fruits.

Apple*: 1 small (2½-inch diameter)

Banana*: 1 small (less than 6 inches long—contains 19 grams of carbohydrates)

Blueberries: ¾ cup

Cantaloupe*: 1 cup cubes or balls

Cherries*: 12

Grapefruit, pink or white*: ½ grapefruit (4-inch diameter)

Grapes: 17 small

Kiwifruit*: 1 large

Mango: ½ small (contains 18 grams of carbohydrates)

Orange*: 1 fresh fruit or ¾ cup mandarins juice-packed canned, drained

Papaya: 1 cup cubes

Peach: 1 medium fresh or ½ cup juice-packed canned

Pear: ½ large fresh or ½ cup juice-packed canned

Pineapple: ¾ cup fresh or ½ cup juice-packed canned (contains 19 grams of carbohydrates)

Plums*: 2 small fresh (2⅛-inch diameter) or 3 dried (prunes)

Pomegranate: ½ cup seeds/juice sacs

Raspberries*: 1 cup fresh

Strawberries*: 1¼ cups whole

Watermelon: 1¼ cups cubes or balls

Fresh Fruit, Season by Season

Here's a list of the varieties of fruit typically available each season, including fruits both grown locally (within 100 miles of you) and imported.

SPRING	SUMMER	FALL	WINTER
Bananas	Cantaloupe	Apples	Apples
Grapefruit	Cherries	Bananas	Bananas
Mangoes	Peaches	Blueberries	Grapefruit
Papaya	Plums	Cranberries	Grapes
Strawberries	Watermelon	Grapes	Kiwifruit
		Pears	Oranges
		Raspberries	

Sweet and Easy Ways to Savor Fruit

If you're not an apple-a-day type, the suggestions below can help you eat fruit more often and enjoy it more, too. Remember to eat fruit as part of a meal to stave off sugar spikes. If you're eating fruit as a snack, pair it with a small amount of protein—say, an ounce of nuts or cheese.

★ Start your day with fruit. Slice a fresh peach onto your cereal, layer berries in a yogurt breakfast parfait, or cut yourself a wedge of fresh melon.

★ To add natural sweetness to your morning oatmeal, add one small chopped pear or apple or half a banana, and let the fruit "cook in."

★ For a quick on-the-run breakfast or snack, top a slice of whole grain toast with a tablespoon of peanut butter and a serving of sliced banana.

★ If you bring your lunch to work, pack a portable fruit—a tangerine, a banana, berries, or grapes. If you buy, hit a local salad bar, which usually offers fresh fruit salad.

★ For lunch, top low-fat cottage cheese with one serving of your fruit of choice.

★ Snack on apple slices spread with peanut butter.

★ Whip up a fruit smoothie for breakfast or lunch. It's easy—just toss a cup of fat-free or low-fat milk or yogurt in the blender, throw in some fresh or frozen berries or a small banana, and hit "blend."

★ Add slices of your favorite fruit to a garden salad for a burst of flavor and nutrients.

★ After dinner, reach for fruit for dessert. Think outside the box— baked apples and poached pears in the winter, cold fruit soups or homemade sorbet in the summer. Log on to prevention.com and scroll through the recipe section—you'll find plenty of recipes.

Boost the Fruit Effect

Now that you know how to maximize the taste of fruit, these strategies can help you maximize its nutritional benefits and convenience.

★ Buy local when you can. The fruit available depends on where you live, but whatever it is, if you hit a roadside stand, the offerings will be cheaper and at the peak of flavor and nutrients.

★ At the supermarket, buy fruit in season (see "Fresh Fruit, Season by Season" on page 108). Winter means citrus— oranges, grapefruit, and tangerines—but you'll find exotic tropical fruit, too.

★ Buy frozen or canned (in water or juice) to have on hand. I prefer frozen, because it's frozen at the peak of its nutrients and isn't doused with syrup of any kind. If mangoes and your favorite berries don't grow in your region or are out of season, chances are you can find them in the frozen-foods section.

★ Some kinds of fruit, particularly apples, seem larger than they were years ago. If yours seems huge, eat one half, cover the other with plastic wrap, and pop it in the fridge for later.

★ Keep "portable fruit" at the office. While pomegranates and pineapple don't fit the bill, apples, pears, and bananas are easy to eat on your way out the door or keep in your desk at the office.

Rescuer No. 8

RED WINE AND ALCOHOL

One glass a day

Though red wine in moderation is part of the traditional Mediterranean diet, alcohol is optional on the Diabetes Rescue Diet. There are good reasons not to drink red wine or any alcohol if it's not already part of your life. You may not care for its taste, effects, or calories. Perhaps you're concerned about its addictive potential, your faith forbids it, or your doctor has advised that you avoid alcohol completely.

So if you don't imbibe now, don't start. But if you do and wonder whether alcohol fits into this diet, the answer is yes—in moderation.

Fact is, scientific research supports moderate drinking. Most prospective studies, which follow large numbers of people over time, show that moderate drinkers have a significantly lower risk of diabetes, compared with nondrinkers. In one 2006 study of more than 35,000 women, those who drank red wine more than once a week reduced their diabetes risk by 16 percent, compared with those who drank it less often, researchers led by the University of Minnesota School of Public Health found. White wine, beer, and liquor were similarly protective. In another study, having less than one drink a day cut diabetes risk by half—great news if you're in the habit of splitting a beer.

Nor does moderate alcohol use appear to harm people with type 2 diabetes who are free of serious conditions like uncontrolled high blood pressure or cholesterol. In a 2008 study, another University of Minnesota team divided 18 people with diabetes into two groups. One group drank 4 to 8 ounces of white wine a day; the other abstained from alcohol. After a month, there was virtually no difference in triglycerides and HDL cholesterol, blood sugar, hemoglobin A1c, and blood pressure between the moderate drinkers and the abstainers. Nor did the moderate drinkers experience hypoglycemic episodes. Actually, those who drank reduced their fasting insulin!

As you'll see, one glass of wine (or even a martini) a day can also do great things for your heart, studies suggest. Moderate alcohol consumption has been found to relax blood vessels, reduce the ability of blood to clot, and help prevent blood fats from forming the blockages in arteries that can cause heart attack and stroke. So if you enjoy a glass of wine or a beer at dinner or a postwork cocktail, you can raise your (one) glass with confidence. Let's look at the evidence more closely.

A Toast to Diabetes Protection

People who drink in moderation typically live healthier lifestyles than either heavy drinkers or teetotalers, research suggests. In a 2010 Dutch study, researchers examined the link between alcohol intake and the incidence of diabetes, following 35,000 people for more than 10 years. These folks were already at low risk for diabetes—they didn't smoke, ate a healthy diet, maintained a healthy weight, and exercised regularly. In those 10 years, 796 people developed diabetes.

Compared with nondrinkers, moderate drinkers were 45 percent less likely to develop diabetes, and the lower risk persisted even when the researchers controlled for other lifestyle factors. For example, when only normal-weight people were analyzed, moderate drinkers were 65 percent less likely to develop diabetes. Among only regular exercisers, moderate drinkers had a 35 percent lower risk. These findings can't be explained by a healthier lifestyle alone, the researchers said—in some way not yet understood, alcohol contributed directly to a lower incidence of diabetes.

But scientists also want to uncork the mysteries of how red wine might help regulate blood sugar. Using test-tube studies, scientists at the University of Massachusetts at Amherst analyzed how well red and white wines suppressed a certain enzyme that triggers the absorption of glucose by the small intestine. Medications currently used to treat diabetes also target this enzyme, called alpha-glucosidase.

Red wines suppressed the enzyme by nearly 100 percent, compared with white wine's 20 percent, and contained roughly 10 times more polyphenol antioxidants, the team found. It may be that red wine's polyphenols curb the activity of alpha-glucosidase and slow

Meet the
MAXIMIZER
Red Wine

The flavonoids in red wine pack a potent antioxidant punch. Researchers at the University of California, Davis, tested a variety of wines to determine which types have the highest concentrations of flavonoids. The study's top three most flavo-ful red wines:

Cabernet Sauvignon

Petit Syrah

Pinot Noir

Merlots and red Zinfandels contain fewer flavonoids, the researchers found. Bottom line: Drier red wines have the highest flavonoid boost. And FYI, the sweeter the wine, the fewer the flavonoids.

Red Protects after Heart Attacks

For those with diabetes who've had heart attacks, one small glass of vino a day may help lessen postattack heart damage, a 2006 study suggests.

People with diabetes have higher levels of system-wide inflammation and cellular damage caused by free radicals (oxidative stress). These problems occur after heart attacks, too, and cause permanent injury to the heart. Might red wine's powerful anti-inflammatory and antioxidant powers be able to help?

To find out, researchers from Italy had 115 people with diabetes who'd suffered heart attacks follow the Mediterranean diet. But one group drank one 4-ounce glass of red wine a day, while another group drank no alcohol at all. Both before the study and 1 year later, the researchers examined certain markers of heart health and oxidative stress. At the end of the study, the wine drinkers had better heart function, as measured by an echocardiogram. They also had lower levels of certain chemicals and proteins that suggest cell damage and system-wide inflammation. Specifically, the wine drinkers had lower levels of nitrotyrosine, C-reactive protein, tumor necrosis factor—alpha, interleukin-6, and interleukin-18.

Several large studies have zeroed in on red wine, specifically, as heart protective, the study noted. For example, in a 2005 analysis of 13 studies and more than 200,000 people published in the medical journal *Circulation,* red wine slashed diabetes risk by 32 percent, compared with beer's 22 percent. (But there's some evidence that white wine may be heart-healthy, too—see "What If I Don't Like . . . Red Wine?" on page 115.)

the passage of carbohydrates into the bloodstream, thereby preventing blood sugar spikes, the study said.

According to a 2011 study, a small glass of red wine a day may work as well as or better than a commonly prescribed diabetes drug, Austrian researchers found. The possible reason: molecules in wine called ligands. These researchers studied how strongly ligands attached to a protein called PPAR-gamma, which helps glucose get into fat cells. Then they compared ligands' ability to bind this protein to that of rosiglitazone (marketed as Avandia). This drug also targets PPAR-gamma in fat cells to make them more sensitive to insulin and help them process glucose.

White wines didn't bind to PPAR-gamma so well, the study found. But the reds! In one test, the tendency of the molecules in about 3.4 ounces of red wine to bind to this protein was up to four times as strong as the same tendency in a daily dose of rosiglitazone.

Red wine contains the potent antioxidants epicatechin gallate (ECG) and ellagic acid, and these two attached to PPAR-gamma the best, the study found. Some of red wine's antidiabetic activity may be due to these powerful antioxidants' activation of PPAR-gamma, the researchers said.

To Your (Heart) Health

My wife and I share a glass of Pinot Noir most days, and for me, red wine is one of the many pleasures of "going Mediterranean." It may also be a heart saver. Evidence suggests that a daily glass of red may help keep fatty deposits from forming in blood vessels, especially in the coronary arteries. These deposits reduce bloodflow to the heart. They may also form clots that block the coronary arteries, resulting in chest pain or even a heart attack.

Red wine, in moderation, also increases "good" HDL cholesterol. That goes for other types of alcohol, too—studies have shown that one to two drinks per day raise HDL by about 12 percent. This extra HDL takes some of the "bad" LDL cholesterol out of circulation and reduces the amount available to form fatty deposits.

Red wine's plant chemicals may help keep blood vessels and arteries clear, too. In the mid-'90s, researchers discovered that red wine contains the powerful antioxidant resveratrol. This find gave rise to the French Paradox: Though the French eat lots of artery-clogging saturated fats (all that cheese and butter!) and smoke like chimneys, they have a surprisingly low rate of heart attack and stroke. It may be that the resveratrol in all that red wine they drink protects their hearts. One Italian study even found that a glass of red wine with a meal may help rid the body of potentially damaging fats before they reach blood vessels.

So if you love red wine, *Salute!* If you don't, moderate consumption of any type of alcohol confers benefits, a pair of scientific reviews published in the same 2011 issue of the *British Medical Journal* found. These reviews, both led by researchers at the University of Calgary in Alberta, analyzed nearly 150 studies on the effects of alcohol consumption on biomarkers associated with heart disease.

The first review, of 63 studies, linked 15 to 30 grams of alcohol a day (one drink for women, up to two for men) to significantly higher levels of HDL, lower levels of fibrinogen (a substance that helps blood to clot), and higher levels of adiponectin and apolipoprotein A1.

The hormone adiponectin is linked with a reduced risk of heart

WHAT IF I DON'T LIKE . . .
RED WINE?

Lift a glass of white. The flesh of grapes is just as heart-healthy as the skin, thanks to other antioxidants in the grapes themselves, a 2006 study showed.

Research has suggested that grapes' heart-healthy benefits come from anthocyanins—antioxidant compounds found mostly in the skins. While red wines are made with both skins and pulp, white wines don't include the skins. That's why red wines, which contain more anthocyanins, are thought to be more heart-protective.

In this study, an American-led team of Italian scientists fed laboratory rats either water or equal amounts of grape flesh (pulp) extract or grape skin extract for 30 days.

The skin and pulp extracts protected the rats from heart attacks equally well, the study found. Compared with the rats that got water, those fed either extract had attacks that were significantly less severe. Further, extracts of both skins and pulp appeared to have the same level of antioxidant activity.

While the skins did contain high levels of anthocyanins, white wine has two potent antioxidants of its own: tyrosol and hydroxytyrosol. Both seem to stop oxidation of LDL cholesterol and reduce inflammation, and both are found in olive oil but not in red wine. It may be that these antioxidants are part of what make white wine—and the Mediterranean diet—so good for the heart, the study said.

disease and diabetes, while apolipoprotein A1 is a major component of HDL. These results were similar for all three types of alcohol evaluated—wine, beer, and spirits.

The significant changes in levels of HDL, fibrinogen, and adiponectin "were well within a pharmacologically relevant magnitude," the study said. In other words, moderate consumption of alcohol provided benefits comparable to those of medications.

In the other review of nearly 150 studies, one drink a day or less (2.5 to 14.9 grams of alcohol a day) cut the risk of death by cardiovascular disease, coronary heart disease, and stroke by 14 to 25 percent. The incidence of both coronary heart disease and stroke was similarly reduced.

A Daily Drink: Easy on the Waist

Nutritionists typically view alcohol as empty calories—and it can be, if you drink to excess. However, a daily serving of wine, beer, or spirits doesn't have to widen your waistline. A 2010 study of almost 20,000 women linked light to moderate alcohol intake with less weight gain, not more.

Specifically, women who drank from 15 to less than 30 grams of alcohol a day (one to two drinks per day) were 30 percent less likely to become overweight, compared with nondrinkers. Those who drank from 5 to less than 15 grams a day were 24 percent less likely.

In the study, researchers from Brigham and Women's Hospital in Boston examined the daily alcohol intake of more than 19,000 women ages 39 and older who were enrolled in the Women's Health Initiative. None of the women were overweight when they entered the study, and all filled out an initial questionnaire about their alcohol consumption.

About 40 percent reported that they did not drink at all, while 33 percent reported consuming the equivalent of about two alcoholic drinks a week. Another 20 percent reported that they had approximately one drink a day, and 6 percent had one to two a day.

Over an average of 13 years of follow-up, most of the women gained some weight. But the self-described nondrinkers gained the most, while moderate drinkers (no more than two a day) gained the least. This remained true even after the researchers factored in variables that influence weight gain, such as age, race, total calorie intake, activity level, and smoking. The conclusion: Women of normal weight who are light to moderate drinkers don't gain excessive amounts of weight.

In another 2005 study of 8,236 men and women, Texas Tech University researchers also found that those who had one to two alcoholic drinks a day were about 30 percent less likely to be overweight than complete abstainers. But those who had four or more drinks a day were 30 and 46 percent more likely to be overweight and obese, respectively.

The results do not suggest that people should drink moderately to lose weight, the researchers noted. Scientists still need to find out how alcohol use might influence weight control. But the findings do suggest that there's no reason to promote complete abstention among those who regularly drink alcohol, the study said.

Drink Smart, Drink Safe

One word that appears over and over in these studies is *moderation*. The studies—and the experts—are pretty clear: If you choose to drink alcohol, drink moderately. If you're a woman, that means one drink a day; if you're a man, two. (No, you can't save them up and drink them all on Saturday night.)

While the evidence that links moderate drinking to heart and diabetes protection is solid, there's equally strong evidence that excessive alcohol use can cause serious health problems, including addiction.

Oil and Water (Turned to Wine) Do Mix

Healthy arteries and blood vessels have flex, which helps your heart move blood through your body. Vessels' ability to flex comes from their inner lining, called the endothelium. Arteries with no "give" in the endothelium raise the risk of high blood pressure and cardiovascular disease.

A daily glass or two of red wine improves the flexibility of arteries' inner lining in both healthy people and those with heart disease, research has found. But in 2008, Greek researchers wanted to know how red wine and another staple of the Mediterranean diet—olive oil—affect endothelium function when they're consumed together.

For 4 days, the researchers fed 15 healthy people a light meal that included just over 8 ounces of either red or white wine and about 3 tablespoons of either extra-virgin or refined olive oil added to vegetable soup. (Made from the first olives of each year's harvest, extra-virgin olive oil is richer in antioxidants than any other type.)

The volunteers consumed the oil and wine in every combination—red wine and either extra-virgin or refined olive oil, and white wine and either extra-virgin or refined olive oil. Then the researchers tested the participants' bloodflow 1, 2, and 3 hours after the meal. The test used, called flow-mediated dilation (FMD), measures how well blood flows through a certain artery. For this study, the researchers measured the FMD of the brachial artery, which runs from shoulder to elbow.

The volunteers' arteries dilated only after the meals with red wine and extra-virgin olive oil, the study found, and these improvements lasted up to 2 hours after the meal, compared with fasting levels. The researchers credited the antioxidants in red wine and extra-virgin olive oil.

Don't drink red wine or any other alcohol if you have a personal or family history of alcohol abuse or liver disease.

The definition of "one drink" is also clear:

★ 5 ounces of wine

★ 12 ounces of beer

★ 1.5 ounces of 80-proof distilled spirits, such as vodka

So if you don't drink now, don't start. But if you have diabetes and choose to imbibe, talk to your doctor or a member of your health team about the guidelines below and whether moderate drinking is right for you. One more thing: If your doctor has advised you not to drink alcohol, follow those orders, period.

★ Never, ever drink to excess. Too much alcohol can cause your blood sugar to drop to dangerous levels.

★ Drink alcohol only with food.

★ Don't drink if your blood sugar is already low. Eat something to raise it before you imbibe.

★ Check your blood sugar more often when you drink. This will help you prevent lows.

★ Avoid sweet wines or cordials, which contain high amounts of sugar.

★ If you have a cocktail, avoid sugar-laden mixed drinks. Order hard spirits with water or diet soft drinks.

★ Alcohol can affect the effectiveness of oral diabetes medications and insulin. If you use insulin or take diabetes meds, talk to your doctor about how alcohol may affect them or other medications you're taking.

★ Consider enjoying your glass of wine or beer or your cocktail after you eat. Alcohol stimulates appetite, and that predinner drink may cause you to overeat, which can affect your blood sugar.

★ Consider wearing a medical ID bracelet or necklace. The symptoms of hypoglycemia can appear similar to those of intoxication.

Rescuer No. 9

DAIRY

Three servings a day

There's a host of reasons for the recent increase in both obesity and diabetes, but here's one you haven't heard—and it could explain a lot.

During the ultrafattening years from 1977 to 1992, the calories consumed in the United States from sweetened beverages well more than doubled, while consumption of dairy products plummeted. Actual stats: Sweet drinks increased 135 percent, while dairy went down 38 percent.

As a result of this one change, the average person wound up taking in 278 more calories a day. Since every extra 10 calories can add a pound when eaten regularly, we're talking major weight gain.

But is it just that soda is bad or that dairy products might actually be important helpers in warding off weight gain and diabetes? Lots of research points to dairy as a major diabetes fighter. Specifically, low-fat dairy, which gives you all the key nutrients in cheese, yogurt, and milk—protein, calcium, magnesium, folate and other B vitamins, vitamin D, and the powerful antioxidant vitamins A and E—without the saturated fat and cholesterol.

The evidence for dairy as a diabetes fighter and cardiovascular champion is so strong that one of the tweaks we've made in converting the traditional Mediterranean diet into the Diabetes Rescue Diet is in the dairy department. While the traditional diet calls for moderate to low dairy consumption, we've gone with moderate to generous. Here's why.

Dairy In, Diabetes Out

A study published in the journal *Diabetes Care* reported on more than 37,000 middle-aged women who were followed for an average of 10 years. Those who were in the top fifth of dairy consumption (2.9 servings a day) were 21 percent less likely to develop diabetes than those who consumed little dairy.

The benefit seemed mostly to come from low-fat dairy, the researchers noted. Women who consumed the most low-fat dairy (about two servings a day) were 31 percent less likely to develop diabetes than those who consumed practically none. And, the researchers said, the protection could not be attributed to different amounts of calcium, vitamin D, fiber, or other factors thought to be protective. Body size was not involved, either.

Dairy cannot be accused of sexual discrimination, because almost exactly the same protection was found for men. In a 12-year study of thousands of male health professionals, those who consumed the most dairy had a 23 percent lower risk of developing diabetes than those who consumed the least. And again, low-fat dairy was given most of the credit.

If you want a good example of how diet can stop diabetes in its tracks, dairy again steps into the spotlight. Insulin resistance syndrome (IRS) is considered the first stage of diabetes. The components of IRS include obesity, glucose intolerance, high blood pressure, and high blood fats. Together, these conditions are a major risk factor for type 2 diabetes and heart disease.

After following thousands of people ages 18 to 30 for 10 years, the authors of a study done at Children's Hospital Boston saw that as dairy consumption went up, every one of the IRS components went down. The young people who ate the most dairy were 72 percent less likely to develop two or more components of IRS.

Interestingly, the researchers also found that this protection was true only for young people who were overweight. Those, of course, are the ones who most need protection from slipping into full-blown diabetes.

Another study, in England, looked at diet and the development of metabolic syndrome, a similar cluster of problems—such as impaired glucose control and a large waist—regarded as a slippery slope that can lead to diabetes. In a group of men ages 45 to 59, researchers found that those who drank a pint or more of milk a day had a 62 percent lower risk of metabolic syndrome. Those who consumed the most dairy products had 56 percent less risk.

Dairy helps Americans head off diabetes at the pass, too. A study conducted at American health centers from coast to coast found that women who like dairy help keep metabolic syndrome and diabetes away. Women who drank the most milk had a 15 percent lower risk, while those who consumed the most dairy products in general had double the protection—a very impressive 34 percent lower risk. In fact, people in the Mediterranean area get most of their dairy from yogurt and cheese, not milk.

Go Low (Fat), Gain Heart Health

There's an antidairy contingent out there that claims that even low-fat dairy products increase heart disease risk. But the evidence for that claim—based on one flawed study—simply isn't there. In fact, stripped of their saturated fat and cholesterol, low-fat dairy foods may actually help protect your heart. They retain nutrients your heart needs, such as calcium and magnesium and the powerful antioxidant vitamins A and E. Substances unique to milk may play a part, too. Consider the evidence that links low-fat dairy to heart health.

Lower blood pressure: High blood pressure is not only a risk factor for developing heart disease but also a common complication of diabetes. Dairy seems to help—to the point of cutting risk in half. In a study of university students in Spain, those in the top 20 percent of low-fat dairy consumption were 54 percent less likely to develop high blood pressure during a 27-month observation period.

Lower cholesterol: Researchers at Kansas and Pennsylvania State Universities had 64 people drink a quart of fat-free milk a day. After a month, those with the highest cholesterol saw their levels drop almost 10 points. That's almost a 7 percent reduction. Since every 1 percent drop in cholesterol translates to a 2 percent reduction in death from heart disease, milk helped these folks reduce their risk of heart attack or stroke by nearly 14 percent.

Lower body weight: Many studies have found that dairy helps control weight. One of the latest, a 2010 study from Israel, looked at dairy and weight loss among overweight diabetes patients. Those in the top third of dairy calcium consumption were nearly 2½ times more likely to lose at least 8 percent of their body weight during weight-loss diets, compared with those who consumed little. A happy difference!

Again, note that these findings are for low-fat dairy. If you eat a lot of full-fat dairy foods, your blood cholesterol will likely rise, and you definitely don't want that. But low-fat dairy foods are a lot tastier than they used to be. So if you only think you don't like low-fat cheese and milk, give them a try. I think you'll be surprised!

How to Do Dairy Right

The evidence suggests that three servings of dairy a day is strongly protective. If you like milk, that's easy math. Ditto for yogurt and dairy desserts such as frozen yogurt and ice cream (and don't forget pudding made with milk). Cheese gets a bit trickier—it depends on whether you choose natural or processed. In general, 1½ ounces of natural cheese or 2 ounces of processed cheese counts as 1 cup.

Each food listed below counts as a single serving of milk, cheese, or yogurt. You won't find cream, sour cream, or cream cheese on the list—they're too low in calcium. But stick to serving sizes, and you can have them on occasion.

- ★ 1 cup yogurt
- ★ 1½ ounces hard cheese, such as Cheddar, mozzarella, or Swiss
- ★ 2 ounces processed cheese, like American
- ★ ⅓ cup shredded cheese
- ★ 2 cups cottage cheese
- ★ ½ cup ricotta cheese
- ★ 1 cup pudding made with milk
- ★ 1 cup frozen yogurt
- ★ 1½ cups ice cream
- ★ 1 cup milk, including lactose-free and lactose-reduced products and fortified soy beverages

Here's the nice thing about dairy: It's flexible. If you don't like milk, you can opt for cheese and yogurt. The only important guideline: Stick mostly to the fat-free or low-fat versions of your favorite dairy foods—"regular" varieties are packed with saturated fat.

If you usually drink whole milk, step down gradually. From whole milk, switch to reduced fat (2%), then low-fat (1%), and finally fat-free (skim). Remember, although you're cutting calories, you're getting the same amount of calcium and other essential nutrients. Also, choose fat-free or low-fat yogurt or milk more often than cheese. They're better sources of potassium and lower in sodium than most cheeses, and milk is fortified with vitamin D.

But the Mediterranean way of eating isn't restrictive. If you can't resist a full-fat cheese like Brie or you love full-fat cottage cheese,

---

Butter versus Cheese: Which Makes the Cut?

Both cheese and butter are packed with saturated fat, the main dietary cause of high blood cholesterol. But while full-fat cheese is allowed on the Diabetes Rescue Diet, we want you to swap butter for olive oil. Why?

Cheeses are eaten liberally in France and Italy, countries with low incidences of diabetes and heart disease. It is possible that cheese may have a "secret ingredient" that works against the saturated fat, pushing down blood cholesterol, suggests a study conducted at the Baker Heart Research Institute in Melbourne, Australia.

Researchers at the institute decided to look into why cheese eaters should be healthier than butter eaters. In a series of tests, they gave volunteers with mildly high cholesterol 40 grams of dairy fat in the form of either butter or Cheddar cheese for several weeks. Picture that as either 10 teaspoons of butter or about 4 ounces of Cheddar.

The butter eaters saw their LDL ("bad") cholesterol rise significantly, but the cheese eaters didn't. Fermented dairy products such as cheese (yogurt, too) may result in a lower blood-cholesterol level than nonfermented dairy products, the researchers suggested. You certainly don't want to eat a quarter pound of full-fat Cheddar a day, but it's nice to know that the occasional nibble won't drive up your cholesterol.

enjoy it on occasion. Just do as the Mediterraneans do and eat a small amount, savoring every bite.

12 Ways to Dairy Up Your Diet

Perhaps you think milk is for kids. Or maybe you're a dairy dropout; you don't have anything against dairy, but apart from cheese, it just doesn't make it into your shopping cart. The tips below will help you add a little to any meal—and it's simpler than you think.

★ If you like milk but drink it only occasionally, commit to drinking a cup with at least one of your daily meals. Buy a quart of 1% milk and go from there. Steam yourself a cup before you go to

Ice Cream: "Can I Have Some? Please?"

Ice cream is obviously not something you should eat every day on the Diabetes Rescue Diet. But as an occasional treat, it might even be good for you. I'll bet you've never heard this before, but a major study of dairy product consumption and health came up with the finding that ice cream actually helps prevent diabetes!

Now I know you're thinking this study must have been done by Dairy Queen or Häagen Dazs, but it wasn't. The researchers were from top medical centers, including Harvard Medical School, the University of California at Los Angeles, and even the US Centers for Disease Control and Prevention. And it was huge, following the diets and health of more than 37,000 women for an average of 10 years.

The chief finding was that low-fat dairy is very strongly linked to a reduced risk of diabetes. But it also found that ice cream made the cut, along with yogurt and skim milk. Specifically, the study shows that women who ate ice cream two or more times a week had 12 percent less risk of developing diabetes than women who indulged less than once a month. In fact, ice cream was associated with less risk of diabetes than drinking skim milk (an 8 percent lower risk)!

What persuades me that this apparent protection is real is the fact that the bed (it will help you sleep). Or mix a cup of hot cocoa or chocolate milk using sugar-free syrup. Soon you might be up to 2 cups a day, and getting that last cup will be that much easier.

★ If you're a fan of coffeehouse drinks, order your cappuccino or latte with fat-free milk. You soon won't notice the difference.

★ Sprinkle a bit of crumbled feta cheese over a mixture of cold cooked lentils, minced red onion, and diced green pepper. Dress with olive oil and vinegar for a delicious cold salad.

★ Choose harder cheeses you can grate, such as Parmesan and Romano, and sprinkle over your dishes. You'll get all the flavor of full-fat cheese with fewer calories and less saturated fat.

medical researchers ruled out some 15 different factors that might distort the results. It wasn't that ice cream eaters were already thinner, or that they exercised more, or that they were younger. Remarkably, researchers even ruled out the preventive benefit from the calcium and vitamin D in ice cream. There is something special about dairy that helps prevent diabetes, and that something is in ice cream, too!

Although the women in the study ate ice cream several times a week, let me remind you that too much ice cream can lead to weight gain. If you're going to dip in now and then, keep the portions small—½ cup—and favor low-fat brands.

The "Healthy" Ice Cream Substitute That Backfires

If you're tempted to try an ice cream substitute from the health food section of your market, be careful. In one study, people with well-controlled type 2 diabetes were given either regular ice cream sweetened with sucrose or a tofu (soybean curd) product sweetened with fructose, which was thought to produce a smaller rise in blood sugar. The researchers were surprised to find that the "healthy" tofu ice cream substitute actually caused a higher spike in blood sugar than the regular stuff! They suspect there were hidden sugars involved.

★ Savor a classic Italian *insalata caprese*—place a slice of tomato atop a slice of part-skim mozzarella. Drizzle with olive oil and crown with a sprig of fresh basil, if possible.

★ Spread cottage cheese on whole grain toast. Sprinkle it with a no-calorie sweetener and a dash of cinnamon, or top with bananas.

★ If you typically make oatmeal with water, use 1% or fat-free milk instead. Do the same thing if you open a can of cream of tomato soup for lunch or dinner.

★ Top your baked potato, quesadilla, taco, soup, or chili with yogurt. Its taste and texture are virtually indistinguishable from sour cream's, especially if you use Greek yogurt, which is thicker and more flavorful.

★ Make the tangy Greek dip *tzatziki*: Line a sieve with cheesecloth, place over a medium bowl, and add 2 cups plain Greek yogurt. Cover and let it drain in the refrigerator overnight. The next day, seed and grate 1 cucumber and place in a small bowl with a little salt. Cover and chill for 3 hours. Transfer the drained yogurt to another bowl. Mix in 2 tablespoons fresh lemon juice, 2 tablespoons dill (fresh, if you can get it), and 1 minced garlic clove. Squeeze the excess liquid from the

Ice Cream versus Cake! Which to Take?

So you're at Cousin Katie's house, and after dinner she triumphantly marches in with a large cake and a bowl of ice cream. As others smile and make plates of chocolate cake à la mode, you go slightly nuts. "I can't refuse both! I'll seem like an ingrate—or an invalid," you think. "But I can't eat both, either—my blood sugar will go up like a rocket. So which should I take? They both look yummy!"

A pair of researchers found the answer to your dilemma. When they compared equal servings of cake and ice cream for their effects on blood sugar, they found that the spikes after ice cream were "much lower." So leave the fork and grab a spoon!

WHAT IF I DON'T LIKE . . .
DAIRY?

Go the supplement route. While some studies show that dairy, rather than its calcium, is the main protector, others suggest calcium supplements may help. In the Nurses' Health Studies, which followed more than 83,000 women for all of 20 years, researchers looked at intakes of calcium and vitamin D from foods and supplements. The conclusion: Getting more than 1,200 milligrams of calcium and more than 800 IU of vitamin D a day was associated with a 33 percent lower risk of developing diabetes, compared with lesser amounts.

Bolstering this finding are results from a different study, carried out at Tufts–New England Medical Center and published in 2007. More than 300 adults were involved, and half took a combination of 500 milligrams of calcium and 700 IU of vitamin D_3, while others took a placebo (a pill with no effect). Three years later, it turned out that the supplements seemed to have a strong protective effect against early stage diabetes for the people who had impaired glucose control at the start of the study.

For these people—at heightened danger of developing diabetes—those who took supplements experienced a tiny rise in fasting blood sugar after 3 years—just 0.4 milligram. Those not taking the supplements saw their fasting sugars go up 6.1 milligrams—15 times as much! And the supplemented group also experienced a much smaller rise in insulin resistance—a classic early sign of diabetes—some 18 times less than the unsupplemented.

cucumber and add to the yogurt. Season with pepper, cover, and chill for at least 2 hours. It's great with toasted pita wedges or whole grain crackers.

★ Add salsa to your cottage cheese—it really takes the flavor up a notch.

★ When was the last time you had real pudding, made with real milk? Prepare some homemade or sugar-free chocolate pudding, using 1% or fat-free milk.

★ Top cut-up fruit with low-fat flavored yogurt for a quick and healthy snack or dessert.

SOURCES OF LOW- AND HIGHER-FAT DAIRY

Wondering which of your favorite dairy foods fit into your diet (and which to splurge on)? This handy-dandy table can help. Clearly, the foods listed toward the bottom of each category are higher in calories, total and saturated fat, and cholesterol. While you don't have to give them up completely, choose lower-fat, lower-cholesterol options most often.

MILK/SOUR CREAM*	CALORIES	TOTAL FAT (G)	SATURATED FAT (G)	CHOLESTEROL (MG)
Milk, fat-free	86	0.5	0.5	0.5
Milk, chocolate, 1%	158	2.5	2	3
Milk, 1%	102	2	2	12
Buttermilk	98	2	1	4
Sour cream (2 Tbsp)	51	5	3	11
Milk, whole	146	8	5	24
Milk, chocolate, whole	208	8	5	30

Based on an 8-ounce serving unless otherwise specified

CHEESE*	CALORIES	TOTAL FAT (G)	SATURATED FAT (G)	CHOLESTEROL (MG)
Mozzarella, fat-free	63	0	0	8
Cottage cheese, 1% (½ cup)	81	1	1	5
Parmesan (1 Tbsp)	22	1	1	15
Cottage cheese, 2% (½ cup)	102	2	1	9
Swiss, low-fat	75	2	1	15
Cheddar, low-fat	74	3	2	9
Colby, low-fat	74	3	2	9
American, low-fat	77	3	2	15
Mozzarella, part-skim, low-moisture	108	7	4	27
Monterey Jack, low-fat	131	9	6	27
Ricotta, skim milk (½ cup)	170	10	6	38

CHEESE*	CALORIES	TOTAL FAT (G)	SATURATED FAT (G)	CHOLESTEROL (MG)
Goat cheese, soft	114	9	6	20
Neufchatel	111	10	6	32
Feta cheese	112	9	6	38
American	141	10	7	27
Provolone	149	11	7	29
Gouda	151	12	7	48
Blue cheese	150	12	8	32
Cheddar	171	14	9	45

Based on a 1.5-ounce serving unless otherwise specified

YOGURT*	CALORIES	TOTAL FAT (G)	SATURATED FAT (G)	CHOLESTEROL (MG)
Yogurt, fat-free, vanilla, low-calorie sweetener	105	0.5	0.5	5
Yogurt, fat-free, plain	137	0.5	0.5	5
Yogurt, whole	149	8	5	32

Based on a 3.5-ounce serving unless otherwise specified

DAIRY DESSERT*	CALORIES	TOTAL FAT (G)	SATURATED FAT (G)	CHOLESTEROL (MG)
Ice cream, vanilla, fat-free	99	0	0	0
Pudding, chocolate, fat-free, ready to eat	110	0.5	0.5	1
Frozen yogurt, chocolate, fat-free, no sugar	77	1	0.5	3
Pudding, chocolate, ready to eat	157	5	1	3
Frozen yogurt, chocolate	115	4	3	4
Ice cream, vanilla	145	8	5	32

Based on a ½-cup serving

Rescuer No. 10

LESS MEAT

*3 ounces or less of red meat a week;
avoid processed meats*

"Beef . . . it's what for dinner," Robert Mitchum used to say in a TV ad. Perhaps he should have added, "Well, maybe once in a while."

One of the chief components of the Mediterranean diet is eating red meat "rarely." But is cutting back on beef and pork really that important for your health—and diabetes in particular?

One notable study, carried out by the National Institutes of Health and the AARP (the retired folks' group), followed an enormous number of people—some half a million—for 7 years. The idea was to discover possible relationships between diet and health outcomes. The results were published in a 2009 issue of *Archives of Internal Medicine*.

One finding: Women who were in the top 20 percent of meat eaters were 31 percent more likely to wind up in the Great Steakhouse in the Sky over those 7 years; men, 36 percent more likely. As for death from heart disease (the greatest immediate threat to people with diabetes), meat-loving women had a 50 percent higher risk. The big-time eaters of both red and processed meat, such as bacon and hot dogs, also had a higher risk of cancer mortality and death from any cause at all.

Now, you might suspect that meat lovers perhaps have other reasons for these health dangers. Maybe they're all too fat or smokers. But no, that's not true. The researchers adjusted the risk for a host of possible "confounders," including body mass index, smoking, age, gender, and physical activity—even the use of vitamin supplements— and the risk from lots of meat was still there.

But what about eating meat and the risk of developing diabetes? A study from health centers in Hawaii, published in *Public Health Nutrition,* found some very incriminating results. Following tens of thousands of people for all of 14 years, the scientists found that women in the top fifth of red-meat eaters were 30 percent more likely to develop diabetes than those who ate the least. Men who most often ate burgers, steaks, ribs, and other kinds of red meat were at a 43 percent higher risk of being diagnosed with diabetes.

People who ate the most processed meats were at even greater risk. Women had a 45 percent higher risk and men, 57 percent higher. It's worth mentioning that intake of fresh poultry was not associated at all with risk of diabetes.

Another important point: This large study was multiethnic, with thousands of Caucasians, Japanese Americans, and native Hawaiian Islanders involved. So it doesn't reflect something unusual about the metabolism of any one group.

The researchers concluded, "Our findings support the growing evidence that red and processed meat intake increases risk for diabetes irrespective of ethnicity and level of body mass index." In other words, it doesn't matter where your ancestors came from or if you're overweight or not—lots of meat makes you more vulnerable to diabetes.

The take-home message? Use meat the way you do mustard or hot sauce: to add flavor. You don't have to stop eating it entirely, and you can cut back gradually, so you won't feel deprived. Your rewards: a healthier heart, better blood sugar, and a slimmer waistline. And the food ain't bad, either.

Less Meat Downsizes Diabetes

Several studies have associated eating lots of red meat with a higher risk of type 2 diabetes—and a high intake of processed meats raises risk even more. For example, in a 37,000-woman study at Brigham and Women's Hospital in Boston, women who ate red meat at least five times a week had a 29 percent higher risk of type 2 diabetes than those who ate it less than once a week. The scientists suspect the cholesterol in red meat is to blame.

But compared with women who ate processed meats less than once a week, those who ate them at least five times a week had a 43 percent higher risk of diabetes! In this case, the suspected culprit was the additives in processed meat.

In one of the latest studies to look at the association between meat intake and diabetes risk, published in the journal *Diabetologia*, researchers from Norway systematically reviewed 12 studies from all over the world to see if they could find evidence of such a link. And find it they did. Compared with those who ate the lowest amounts of red meat, those who ate the most had a 21 percent increased risk of diabetes. And those who ate the most processed meat increased their likelihood of developing diabetes by 41 percent!

Meat's high content of total and saturated fat could contribute to overweight and obesity—an important risk factor in diabetes, the study noted. However, it may be that the high iron content of red meat reduces insulin's effectiveness or damages the cells that produce insulin.

More studies still have found a link between a diet high in red meat and a heightened risk of metabolic syndrome. Doctors know that this cluster of symptoms—which include obesity, high blood pressure, impaired glucose control, and a large waist—can lead not only to diabetes but also to cardiovascular disease.

In an attempt to understand the relationship between what people eat and the risk of developing metabolic syndrome, researchers at the

Bacon Can Fry Your Health

Some researchers have noticed a stronger connection between diabetes and processed meats, like bacon and hot dogs, than red meat. One study done at Harvard found that the worst of the lot was bacon. Big bacon eaters had a 73 percent higher risk of developing diabetes than noneaters of bacon! Hot dog lovers had a 49 percent higher risk.

Another study concluded that women who eat processed meat five or more times a week had a 91 percent greater risk of developing diabetes than women who ate it less than once a week. For red meat, the risk was just 44 percent higher.

On the face of it, that's surprising. Processed meats contain, on average, similar amounts of saturated fat and not as much cholesterol and iron as red meats. However, processed meat contains significantly more sodium than fresh red meat. It may be that salt's effect on blood pressure weakens blood vessels, research suggests. Further, the nitrates in processed meats may also reduce insulin secretion and impair control of blood sugar, which raises the risk of heart disease and diabetes.

Besides bacon and hot dogs, processed meats include bologna, sausage, pepperoni, and most deli meats. At the very least, don't order a *bacon* cheeseburger! The best bet is to avoid processed meat entirely. Except, of course, for a doggie on the Fourth of July.

University of Minnesota assessed the diets of more than 9,500 middle-aged people. The study was published in the medical journal *Circulation*.

At the start of the study, the researchers suspected that a "prudent" diet of dairy, whole grains, and fruits and vegetables (does this sound familiar?) would lower the risk of metabolic syndrome, while eating a Western-style diet of meat, refined grains, fried foods, and sweetened drinks would raise it.

They were right, and meat was a big factor. In the 9 years the researchers followed the participants, 3,782 of them developed metabolic syndrome. Compared with those who stuck to two servings of meat a week, those who ate two or more servings of meat a day increased their risk of metabolic syndrome by 17 to 26 percent.

Less Red Meat, More Heart Health

In 1984, a classic study of more than 25,000 California Seventh-Day Adventists linked daily meat consumption with a 70 percent greater risk of fatal heart disease in men and a 37 percent greater risk in women. Since the publication of that now-famous study, other research has reached the same conclusion: Big red-meat eaters tend to have a greater risk of dying of heart disease and other diseases like cancer than those who don't.

In a 2009 study, a team headed by the National Cancer Institute examined the link between meat intake and the risk of death in almost 550,000 men and women ages 50 to 71. The team divided the participants into five groups, based on daily intake of red and processed meats. Here are the median highest and lowest intakes the 10-year study found, adjusted for a 2,000-calorie-a-day diet.

Daily Red Meat Intake

Lowest: slightly more than ½ ounce (0.69 ounce)

Highest: 4.4 ounces a day

Daily Processed Meat Intake

Lowest: about 0.11 ounce

Highest: about 1.5 ounces (about 2 slices of deli turkey)

The men who ate the most meat had a 27 percent higher risk of heart disease death and a 22 percent higher risk of cancer death, compared with men who ate the least. Among women, the heaviest meat eaters had a 50 percent higher risk of dying of heart disease—wow!—and a 20 percent higher risk of dying of cancer than women who ate the least meat.

The good news: White meat—including fish, chicken, and turkey—appeared to be protective. Those who ate the most had slightly lower risks of overall and cancer deaths.

The team's conclusion contained a powerful statistic: Limiting red meat to the amount eaten by the lowest-intake group could have reduced heart disease deaths in men by 11 percent and in women by 21 percent.

Here's some cheerier news: Doctors at Harvard figured out that replacing just one daily serving of meat with other protein sources could make a big difference in your risk of coronary heart disease. Replace that burger with chicken and your risk dips by 19 percent. Have fish instead of spareribs and your heart risk drops by all of 24 percent!

The New Normal: Meat as a Treat

If you're the average American, you eat about 120 pounds of beef and pork a year. That's well over 2 pounds of red meat every week—from four to eight servings, depending on portion size.

If that sounds like you, get ready to go Mediterranean and enjoy red meat as a treat, just like the occasional cookie or scoop of ice cream. Based on studies of this ultrahealthy (and delicious) diet, the Diabetes Rescue Diet recommends that if you eat red meat, have a small serving—roughly 3 ounces—once a week, and eat no processed meats at all.

If you choose to splurge on a weekly burger or chop, opt for the leanest cut. Regardless of the kind of meat, cuts with the word *loin* tend to be the leanest. So put sirloin tip steak and top sirloin in your grocery cart. Lean cuts of pork include tenderloin, loin roasts, loin chops, and bone-in rib chops. As for lamb, loin chops and cuts from the shank half of the leg are the leanest cuts you'll find. However, lamb contains roughly two to three times the saturated and unsaturated fats of beef, so save it for a special treat.

If you buy beef, check the US Department of Agriculture grading. Beef labeled "prime" is the top grade but also highest in fat. Most supermarkets sell beef that is graded as "choice" or "select." For the leanest red meat, look for a select grade. (See "Select the Skinniest Beef" on page 138.)

Prepare your lean cuts in healthy ways, too. For example, cut off any visible, solid fat before cooking, and then remove any fat you see before you eat your meat. Finally, after you cook the beef, chill its juices

Select the Skinniest Beef

Although you'll eat less beef on the Diabetes Rescue Diet, it's important to choose the leanest cuts possible—either "extra lean" or "lean." According to government guidelines, beef is considered extra lean if a 3.5-ounce serving contains less than 5 grams of total fat, 2 grams or less of saturated fat, and less than 95 milligrams of cholesterol. Extra-lean cuts of beef include:

- Eye of round roast or steak
- Bottom round roast and steak
- Sirloin tip side steak
- Top sirloin steak
- Top round roast and steak
- 95% lean ground beef

Beef is considered lean if that 3.5-ounce serving contains less than 10 grams of total fat, 4.5 grams or less of saturated fat, and less than 95 milligrams of cholesterol. Lean cuts of beef include:

- Round tip roast and steak
- Top loin (strip) steak
- Round steak
- Flank steak
- Chuck shoulder pot roast
- Tenderloin roast and steak
- Sirloin tip center roast and steak
- T-bone steak
- Chuck shoulder steak

so that you can skim off the hardened fat. Then add the juice to stews, soups, and gravy. (Use these same tips when you prepare and cook your poultry, too—breaded, fried chicken just won't cut it!) Drain the fat from ground meat or poultry in a strainer or colander, rinse the meat with hot water, and then blot it with a paper towel to remove the water.

A word about ground beef: Because hamburgers are cheaper and quicker to cook than roasts or steaks, 40 percent of all the beef we consume is now ground. Yet it contributes more than 60 percent of the saturated fat we get from beef. Switch from a typical (quarter pound) burger to a ground turkey breast burger and you'll dodge more than a third of a day's saturated fat!

Miss Meat? Go Poultry!

If you're used to having bacon or sausage for breakfast, submarine sandwiches at lunch, and pork or beef for dinner, cutting back on red meat may seem daunting. But poultry—chicken, turkey, even game birds—can fill that gap. Who doesn't like a falling-off-the-bone leg of roasted chicken? Or a chicken breast poached in white wine and herbs? Not only does poultry contain less total and saturated fat, research suggests that people with type 2 diabetes who swap red meat for poultry may reap health benefits.

In a 2005 study of 4,304 diabetes-free men and women ages 40 to 69, researchers from Finland found that, compared with those in the lowest quartile of poultry intake, those in the highest had a whopping 30 percent reduced risk of diabetes! The beneficial effect of chicken compared with red meat could be related to lower saturated fat and a higher percentage of polyunsaturated fatty acids, the researchers suggested.

A more-poultry, less-red-meat diet may also reduce the risk of microalbuminuria, a predictor of end-stage kidney failure and an independent risk factor for coronary artery disease, the main cause of death in people with type 2 diabetes. (In microalbuminuria, the kidneys leak small amounts of protein, or albumin.)

In a small study conducted in Brazil, 17 people with type 2 diabetes and large amounts of albumin in their urine randomly followed three different diets for 4 weeks each, with 4-week intervals between each diet: their usual diet, which included red meat; a chicken diet, in which all the usual meat was replaced with dark chicken (skinless leg quarter); and a vegetarian, low-protein diet. All the diets contained at least 50 percent less of the participants' usual protein intake. Replacing red meat with that skinless leg quarter reduced the amount of albumin participants excreted in their urine by 36 percent! The balance of fats in their blood also improved.

The Savory Secret to Healthier Grilling

You may not want to believe it, but those juicy steaks or burgers you grill on a beautiful day are a health risk beyond that caused by their content of saturated fat or cholesterol. That's because when meat is heated to a very high temperature (as with grilling or frying), cancer-causing substances called heterocyclic amines, or HCAs, are formed. HCAs aren't choosy—they'll form on poultry and fish, too.

But you can fight back by marinating beef, poultry, and fish and stirring in antioxidant-rich spices, research suggests.

In a 2008 study, scientists at Kansas State University marinated beef round steaks for an hour in three different store-bought marinades—Caribbean, Southwest, and herb. Steaks were then grilled at 400°F for 5 minutes on each side.

Then the meat was tested for total HCAs. The steak cooked in the Caribbean marinade had an 88 percent reduction in HCAs. Those cooked in the herb and Southwest marinades had a 72 and 57 percent drop in the compounds, respectively.

Commonly available spice-containing marinades can be effective inhibitors of HCA formation and provide reduced exposure to some of the carcinogens formed during grilling, the study said. You can also add antioxidant spices to your own marinades—rosemary, thyme, and turmeric are particularly potent, the study noted. In fact, seasoning beef with rosemary before grilling has been found to reduce HCAs by 30 to 100 percent!

By the way, in keeping with the Diabetes Rescue Diet, consider marinating your meat or poultry in red wine, too. Six hours of marinating in red wine (or beer) cut levels of two types of HCA in beefsteak by up to 90 percent, compared with unmarinated steak, according to a 2008 study conducted in Portugal.

Marinades are an important part of the Rescue Recipes in this book, as well. Try the Grilled Chicken Milanese (page 196) or Grilled Fish and Vegetable Kebabs (page 213) to see how it's done.

You can eat roughly 3 ounces of boneless, skinless chicken a day, either white or dark meat—the same amount the participants in the study ate. If you've never been a big poultry fan, check out the recipes to discover—or rediscover—just how tasty it can be. (The Rescue Recipes start on page 161.) The trick is to prepare poultry with low-fat sauces, rubs, and marinades, which add flavor without fat, and cook it in the same healthy ways you do other meat.

Here's just one example: Marinate chicken breasts in fresh lime juice, sliced green onions, salt, and pepper juice for 3 to 4 hours. Then grill it and top with fresh salsa. (Make the salsa yourself or buy the ready-made kind in the produce aisle of your supermarket.) Use the leftovers for chicken salad the next day. Quick, simple, delicious—and a diabetes-friendly way to satisfy your carnivorous cravings.

Minimum Meat, Maximum Taste

I asked my wife how often we eat red meat. I thought it was once a week. She thought for a moment and estimated it was more like twice a month, usually in chili. Which of course, has lots of healthy beans, tomatoes, and onions.

We used to eat quite a bit more—veal chops, spareribs, rib eye, and meat loaf. But we've slowly shifted away from all that meat and switched to lots more fish, chicken, pasta, bean-filled dishes, and vegetarian stews and soups.

I don't miss meat at all. It may be hard to imagine not eating a juicy steak, burger, or chop every day. But once you take the plunge, you'll see that it's not as tough as you think. These tips can help you change your carnivorous ways.

Don't sideline those veggies. Don't try to eat all your veggies as side dishes. To that end, try this Greek stew, called *ladera*. Boil a pound of frozen green beans for 3 minutes and drain. Sauté a chopped onion in olive oil and add a can of crushed tomatoes, a pinch of sugar, and some parsley. Cook for 10 minutes, add the beans, and simmer for 20 minutes. Top with feta cheese and serve with whole grain bread.

Change up, branch out. As you focus on familiar favorites, try to branch out and think outside the box. Pasta with pesto or topped with

WHAT IF I LOVE ...

RED MEAT?

Then you're a normal, red-blooded American! There are very few Americans who don't love burgers, steaks, ribs, and roasts. So if you're worried about giving up red meat cold turkey (pardon the pun), relax. You don't have to. You can do it gradually with a "step-down" approach. Here's a sample 4-week step-down program.

If you now eat red meat or processed meat every day, cut it back to every other day for 2 weeks. To gauge the right amount, look at your palm. How much meat could it hold? About 6 ounces, as it turns out. Your portion of meat should fit in your palm and last throughout the day. In other words, of that amount, you could eat half for lunch and half for dinner.

Then, for another 2 weeks, gradually step down to the amount that fits in half your palm. Eat it at one meal, added to a variety of dishes, then eat the leftovers at your next meal or the next day. Do that once a week.

Many cuisines use just this tiny portion of meat to flavor a dish made mainly of vegetables, whole grains, and beans. Two examples: the classic Asian stir-fry or Spanish paella. Focus on your favorite nonmeat dishes, such as pasta and bean burritos. Adjust your favorite soup and casserole recipes, too. Add veggies and/or grains; reduce beef, ham, or sausage.

And don't forget, the Diabetes Rescue Diet encourages you to eat fish and poultry. Before long, you'll miss red meat less and look forward to a juicy salmon steak or some savory roasted chicken.

chunky ratatouille, cold gazpacho, baba ghannouj, toasted pita wedges spread with hummus paired with a small chunk of feta, even the perfect PB&J (see "What If I Don't Like ... Nuts?" on page 69) are some tasty options for breakfast, lunch, or even dinner.

Beat a burger craving. Instead of beef, try a broiled marinated portobello mushroom or grilled chicken breast on a crusty roll, or a ground chicken or turkey breast burger.

Try meat substitutes. Veggie burgers, "chicken" nuggets, and hot dogs made with soy are a lot tastier than they used to be. You'll find them in the organic frozen-foods or refrigerated section of your supermarket.

Do mock deli meats. Can't live without pepperoni or lunchmeat? Look for these tasty substitutes, found in the produce section or cold case of most supermarkets.

★ *Tofurky Peppered Deli Slices:* Five slices provide 3 grams of fiber with no saturated fat or cholesterol—and it's just as spicy as the real thing.

★ *Field Roast Lentil Sage artisan deli slices:* The flavor is rich with sage and garlic—heaven for 104 calories per serving.

★ *Yves Meatless Roast without the Beef:* You'll love the texture, and it's a great corned beef substitute for a veggie Reuben.

Build convenience into nonmeat fare. Whipping up veggie, bean, and grain-based dishes can be just as simple as pan-frying a steak or chop—if you plan ahead. Make a slow cooker full of beans on Saturday night and reheat as needed, or go for canned beans. (I love the canned Tex-Mex beans.) Reheat cooked grains for breakfast. Quinoa is delicious as a hot breakfast "cereal" with a bit of low-fat milk or a dollop of low-fat yogurt, cinnamon, and nuts. Frozen veggies are easy to build a meal around, too.

Declare a blackout on meat at certain meals. One rule might be "no meat at breakfast," which will automatically knock out processed meats like bacon and sausage. Then you can flavor your dinner with a bit of red meat or order a small portion when you're out to dinner.

Dine out with less red meat. When you're out to lunch, opt for *salade niçoise*, if it's on the menu, or a Greek salad topped with grilled chicken. Or order from the salad, soup, and appetizer options, which tend to be less meat-centric. At dinner, order a fish dish or share a steak, since the portion will likely be larger than you need anyway.

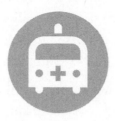

The Rescue Meal Plan and Score Sheet

The following 2 weeks of recipes meet all the criteria for the Diabetes Rescue Diet, yet they are so delicious and easy to follow that you'll never feel like you are limited by a program. Feel free to mix and match meals, or switch out your snack for a dessert or vice versa (you get to have one or the other each day). Whether you use these meal plans or set off on your own, keep track of your Rescuers by using the handy score sheet at the end of the chapter.

Two things to keep in mind:

★ All side dish salads are tossed with a variation of Rescue Vinaigrette (see recipes on page 219).

★ You can choose to enjoy one or two glasses of red wine with dinner instead of having a dessert or snack.

DAY NO. 1

Breakfast

Almond French Toast with Strawberries (page 169)

6 ounces 0% Greek yogurt with ½ cup diced mango or peach and 2 tablespoons sliced natural almonds

Lunch

Baby spinach leaves topped with ½ cup three-bean salad and 2 ounces feta cheese

2 ounces part-skim mozzarella, sliced tomato, and fresh basil sandwich on whole grain roll

Sliced apple

Dinner

Green salad with roasted peppers

2 ounces roast turkey breast

1 cup steamed green beans tossed with ¼ cup diced tomato

Pineapple Roasted Sweet Potatoes (page 226)

Dessert

Flourless Chocolate Cake with Coconut Topping (page 242)

DAY NO. 2

Breakfast

¾ cup muesli

1 cup 1% milk

½ cup banana slices with ½ cup blueberries and ½ ounce chopped walnuts

Lunch

Cucumber, tomato, and baby arugula salad topped with ⅓ cup white beans (cannellini)

English Muffin Pizza (page 186)

Dinner

Chopped tomato and green olive salad

Linguine "Bolognese" (page 199)

Broccoli rabe sautéed with garlic in extra-virgin olive oil

Dessert

Raspberry-Almond Cheesecake (page 240)

DAY NO. 3

Breakfast

1 small apple, sliced and spread with 2 tablespoons nut or seed butter (such as peanut, sunflower, or almond butter)

Strawberry milk: 1 cup 1% milk blended with 1 cup hulled strawberries

Lunch

Chopped green pepper, red onion, tomato, and cilantro salad

Poblano Chile and Bean Soup (page 193)

Snack

6 ounces yogurt

1 cup mixed fruit

Dinner

Arugula salad with ½ cup grapefruit sections

Brown Rice–Stuffed Peppers (page 198)

DAY NO. 4

Breakfast

Steel-Cut Oats with Almonds and Dates (page 166)

¼ cantaloupe eaten off the rind; or 1 cup cubed

1 cup 1% milk

Lunch

Green salad topped with ½ cup mixed berries, 2 tablespoons chopped walnuts, and 2 ounces feta cheese

1 slice toasted whole grain or pumpernickel bread brushed with olive oil

Dinner

Green salad with 1 cup asparagus pieces, ⅓ cup kidney beans, and fresh dill

Oven-Fried Tilapia (page 209)

½ cup roasted new potatoes

Dessert

1 peach, halved and topped with ½ cup part-skim ricotta cheese and 2 teaspoons chopped pistachios

DAY NO. 5

Breakfast

Whole grain English muffin with nut or seed butter

6 ounces 0% Greek yogurt with 1 cup mixed berries

Lunch

Pasta Salad with Tuna, Eggs, and Red Beans (page 182)

½ cup roasted pepper slices with 2 ounces part-skim mozzarella

1 sliced pear

Snack

1 ounce goat cheese on 2 rye crackers with ½ cup baby carrots

Dinner

Mixed green salad with white beans (cannellini), ripe olives,
and green bell peppers

Tomato soup

Grilled Portobello Burgers (page 202)

DAY NO. 6

Breakfast

Sun-Dried Tomato Scramble (page 174)

½ cup banana slices with 1 tablespoon almonds

1 cup 1% milk

Lunch

Roasted Beet, Apple, and Walnut Salad (page 181)

1 slice toasted whole grain or pumpernickel bread brushed with olive oil

Dinner

Romaine lettuce with ½ cup artichoke hearts and ⅓ cup chickpeas

2 ounces roast chicken

1 cup steamed broccoli and cauliflower mix

⅓ cup cooked brown or wild rice

Dessert

1 large sliced plum with ⅓ cup vanilla frozen yogurt and 2 teaspoons chopped pistachios

DAY NO. 7

Breakfast

6 ounces 0% Greek yogurt topped with ½ cup peach slices, ½ cup muesli, and 2 tablespoons sliced natural almonds

Lunch

Chopped cucumber, tomato, and green onion salad

Tomato Lentil Soup (page 190)

1 slice toasted whole grain or pumpernickel bread brushed with olive oil

Dinner

Spinach salad with ½ cup orange sections and 1 tablespoon chopped walnuts

Noodle-Free Eggplant Lasagna (page 200)

Whole grain garlic bread

Dessert

Strawberry-Banana Crepes (page 241)

DAY NO. 8

Breakfast

Multigrain Pancakes with Apple-Raisin Topping (page 164)

½ cup orange sections

1 cup 1% milk

Lunch

Green bean and tomato salad

1 slice open-face grilled (or broiled) cheese sandwich on whole grain bread with 2 ounces shredded reduced-fat Cheddar or Swiss cheese

1 cup watermelon or cantaloupe chunks

Dinner

Tomato salad with ⅓ cup white beans (cannellini) and basil

Roasted Pork Tenderloin and Peppers with Arugula Pesto (page 218)

½ cup cooked whole grain pasta tossed with 1 teaspoon extra-virgin olive oil

Dessert

Panna Cotta with Berries (page 247)

DAY NO. 9

Breakfast

Italian Peppers and Eggs on Toast (page 173)

1 cup pineapple chunks

1 cup 1% milk

Lunch

2 cups mixed fruit salad with 1 ounce (2 tablespoons) chopped walnuts

6 ounces low-fat yogurt

Dinner

Arugula, asparagus, and artichoke salad with 2 ounces feta cheese

1 cup lentil soup

1 slice toasted whole grain bread brushed with 1 teaspoon extra-virgin olive oil

Dessert

Grapefruit and Pomegranate Granita (page 249)

DAY NO. 10

Breakfast

Apple-Cheddar Melt (page 170)

1 cup strawberries

1 cup 1% milk

Lunch

Shredded lettuce with sliced snow peas and radishes

Cold Asian Noodle Salad (page 178)

1 cup watermelon or cantaloupe chunks

Snack

Peach-Almond Frostie (page 237)

Dinner

Butter Beans in Fresh Tomato Sauce (page 220)

Wilted Garlicky Greens (page 222)

½ cup roasted pepper with 2 ounces sliced part-skim mozzarella

DAY NO. 11

Breakfast

¾ cup cold cereal with ½ cup blueberries and 2 tablespoons almonds

1 cup 1% milk

Lunch

Turkey Salad Plate (page 183)

1 cup pineapple chunks

Snack

Hummus (page 231)

Celery sticks

Dinner

Green salad with tomato and avocado

Cheese Polenta with Mushrooms (page 204)

Roasted Peppers with Capers and Anchovies (page 224)

2 thin slices whole grain Italian bread or baguette

DAY NO. 12

Breakfast

Breakfast Biscuit with Fruit Spread (page 167)

6 ounces 0% plain Greek yogurt

1 small banana

Lunch

Root Vegetable Soup (page 191)

Baby spinach salad with 1 sliced pear, 2 ounces reduced-fat Swiss cheese, and 1 tablespoon chopped walnuts

Dinner

Salad of romaine hearts with sliced red onion and ripe olives

Nut-Crusted Chicken Fingers (page 195)

½ cup black beans mixed with ½ cup cherry tomatoes, halved, and ¼ cup corn kernels with basil, served warm or cold

Dessert

Orange-Pineapple Ambrosia (page 243)

DAY NO. 13

Breakfast

½ cup hot cereal with ½ cup raspberries and 2 tablespoons sliced natural almonds

1 cup 1% milk

Lunch

Tabbouleh with Chickpeas and Artichoke Hearts (page 179)

1 ounce reduced-fat cheese

1 cup grapes

Dinner

Spinach salad with broccoli, mushrooms, and red bell pepper

Tomato and Olive Roasted Fish (page 208)

⅓ cup cooked brown or wild rice

Dessert

Roast Pears with Mascarpone Cream (page 244)

DAY NO. 14

Breakfast

Breakfast Biscuit with Fruit Spread (page 167)

6 ounces 0% plain Greek yogurt topped with 1 cup pineapple chunks and 2 tablespoons chopped walnuts

Lunch

Watercress, cucumber, and tomato salad

Crustless Zucchini Quiche (page 189)

1 slice toasted whole grain bread brushed with 1 teaspoon extra-virgin olive oil

Snack

Pita Scoops (page 230)

Dinner

2 cups greens topped with 1 cup three-bean salad

1 slice pizza, plain or with vegetable topping

Your Diabetes Rescue Diet Score Sheet

Want to know how you're doing on the Diabetes Rescue Diet? Use this simple scoring system, based on those used by the researchers who found all the health benefits that flow from sticking to the Mediterranean diet. You'll note that it doesn't ask you to avoid carbohydrates, starchy foods, or fats or stick to a tiny number of calories. This emphasis on the positive is used in all the research-based scoring systems, so we stuck to it!

The Diabetes Rescue Diet is different from the Mediterranean diet in only a few respects. Low-fat dairy is not limited to one serving a day but eaten moderately—because tons of research shows that low-fat dairy is connected with much less incidence of type 2 diabetes and other health problems. Exercise is not included on all Mediterranean diet scores, but it is here. Likewise, not smoking is not on the traditional scores, but it is here, because smoking tremendously increases the risk of diabetes and its complications, regardless of other health habits.

Getting a good score is easier than you think! Keep in mind that the single greatest source of calories in the American diet is soda—which is definitely *not* on the plan. Right away, that opens up a chance to eat more of the good stuff—a handful of nuts, say. And if you don't like fish or wine, you can still score high by eating more salads.

Yes, there are certain foods you should minimize. For example, avoid breakfasting on pancakes with butter and syrup and a side of bacon, and try not to stop for a Whopper, fries, and Coke. That being said, the Diabetes Rescue Diet is more flexible than most other eating plans, which may prohibit all bread, cereal, pasta, beans—even peas!—or added fats like olive oil.

It's easy to whip up an absolutely delicious gourmet meal on your new eating plan, whether you feature American, Italian, French, or Greek cooking—or any combination of cuisines. And when you say "To your health!" or *"Salute!"* those words will be absolutely true!

You'll find the score sheet on the next page. Make photocopies, and mark your score every day until you get the hang of it. Whenever you want to check in, simply make as many copies as you need.

The Score Sheet

Check off the items you've fulfilled, giving yourself 1 point for each. Aim for 10 or more points a day.

The Rescuers

- ☐ Vegetables (4 or more servings)
- ☐ Fruit (3 or more servings)
- ☐ Whole grains (bread, cereal, pasta, brown rice, corn—3 to 4 servings)
- ☐ Beans (1 or more servings)
- ☐ Fish, seafood (1 serving)
- ☐ Nuts (1 serving)
- ☐ Dairy, low-fat (2 to 3 servings)
- ☐ Olive oil, extra-virgin (3 to 4 tablespoons)
- ☐ Red wine (optional) (1 to 2 glasses; if more, score 0)

Extra Points

- ☐ Green salad, vinaigrette
- ☐ Exercise, such as walking
- ☐ No red meat, bacon, or hot dogs
- ☐ No smoking

What's Your Score?

Now total your points for the day. If you scored . . .

10 or more points: Excellent job—you've really taken to eating the Mediterranean way! (Hopefully you're taking your daily walk, too.) If you managed to score extra points, all the better.

8 or 9 points: Very good! One more serving of veggies here, a serving of fish or seafood there, and you've got it down. An easy way to rack up an extra point: Have a salad with vinaigrette dressing at lunch or dinner.

6 or 7 points: Good! You're making steady progress, and that's what we're looking for. Each week, try to add one more point. Pack a piece of fruit for lunch one week, snack on a serving of nuts the next, take your daily walk . . . you'll be racking up those points in no time.

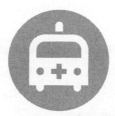

The Rescue Recipes

Here are more than 80 mouthwatering, simple-to-make meals that will rescue you from diabetes and its complications while satisfying your need for taste, comfort, and delight.

Sugar Substitute Basics

We call for a little sugar, maple syrup, or honey in some of our recipes. (As long as you stay within a healthy overall carb count, sugar is safe for people with diabetes.) These small amounts are interchangeable with each other, so, for instance, if you prefer honey over sugar in a recipe, you can substitute it measure for measure. But if you prefer alternative sweeteners, here's how to convert some commonly used commercial products.

SPLENDA

1 tablespoon sugar = 1 tablespoon (or 1½ packets) Splenda

1 tablespoon sugar = 1½ teaspoons Splenda Sugar Blend

1 tablespoon brown sugar = 1½ teaspoons Splenda Brown Sugar Blend

TRUVIA (Stevia)

1 tablespoon sugar = 1¼ teaspoons Truvia

¼ cup sugar = 1 tablespoon + 2 teaspoons Truvia

PURE VIA (Stevia)

1 tablespoon sugar = ¾ teaspoon (or 1½ sachets) Pure Via

¼ cup sugar = 1 tablespoon (or 6 sachets) Pure Via

Multigrain Pancakes with Apple-Raisin Topping

Prep Time: 15 minutes ★ **Total Time:** 45 minutes

You can substitute peaches, pears, or fresh apricots for the apples in the topping and use any chopped, dried fruit in place of raisins. You can also freeze leftover pancakes and topping to have on hand for a quick breakfast at a later time.

Topping

- 1 tablespoon extra-virgin olive oil
- 3 large apples, such as Delicious, cored and thinly sliced
- 1 cup chopped walnuts
- $\frac{1}{3}$ cup raisins
- 1 tablespoon honey (optional)

Pancakes

- $\frac{3}{4}$ cup all-purpose flour
- $\frac{1}{2}$ cup whole wheat flour
- $\frac{1}{2}$ cup quick-cooking oats
- $\frac{1}{4}$ cup fine cornmeal
- $1\frac{1}{2}$ tablespoons baking powder
- $\frac{3}{4}$ teaspoon salt
- 1 egg
- 1 cup low-fat plain yogurt
- 1 cup 1% milk
- 2 tablespoons extra-virgin olive oil
- 2 tablespoons honey

1. *To make the topping:* Heat the oil in a medium saucepan over medium-low heat. Cook the apples, walnuts, and raisins for 5 minutes, stirring often, or until the apples are tender. Stir in the honey (if using). Cover and set aside while making the pancakes.

2. *To make the pancakes:* In a large bowl, whisk together the all-purpose flour, whole wheat flour, oats, cornmeal, baking powder, and salt. Add the egg, yogurt, milk, oil, and honey. Whisk just until smooth.

3. Lightly coat a large skillet or griddle with cooking spray. Place over medium heat.

4. Drop the batter into the skillet by scant ¼ cupfuls. Cook each pancake on 1 side for 3 minutes, or until the pancake is puffed, its edges are cooked, and bubbles start to form on top. Turn and cook for 2 minutes, or until the underside is lightly browned.

5. Serve the pancakes warm with the topping.

Makes 12 (4") pancakes and about 3 cups topping

Per serving: 215 calories, 5 g protein, 26 g carbohydrates, 11 g total fat, 1.5 g saturated fat, 4 g fiber, 379 mg sodium

Steel-Cut Oats with Almonds and Dates

Prep Time: 10 minutes ★ **Total Time:** 35 minutes + soaking time

Toast the oats and almonds the night before, soak overnight, and enjoy quicker-cooking, hearty whole grain oats for breakfast the next day. Traditionally, steel-cut oats are served with a dollop of yogurt or a bit of buttermilk stirred in.

3 **cups water**	½ **cup evaporated 2% milk**
1 **tablespoon light olive oil**	¼ **teaspoon salt**
1 **cup steel-cut oats**	⅓ **cup chopped dates**
1 **cup chopped or sliced natural almonds**	¼ **cup maple syrup (optional)**

1. Bring the water to a boil in a medium saucepan.

2. Heat the oil in a large saucepan over medium-low heat. Cook the oats and almonds, stirring often, for 2 to 3 minutes, or until just golden and fragrant. Remove from the heat and stir in the water. Cover and set aside to cool completely. Refrigerate overnight.

3. The next morning, stir in the milk and salt. Heat to a boil over medium heat. Reduce the heat to low, cover, and simmer for 15 minutes, or until the oats are soft and creamy. Stir in the dates and syrup (if using) and serve.

Makes 4 servings

Per serving: 371 calories, 14 g protein, 46 g carbohydrates, 18 g total fat, 2 g saturated fat, 8 g fiber, 188 mg sodium

Breakfast Biscuits with Fruit Spread

Prep Time: 15 minutes ★ **Total Time:** 25 minutes

Spread these tender biscuits with mashed fresh fruit instead of jelly or jam.

Biscuits

- 1½ cups whole wheat flour
- ½ cup all-purpose flour
- 1 tablespoon baking powder
- ½ teaspoon salt
- ¾ cup low-fat plain yogurt
- ½ cup part-skim ricotta cheese
- ¼ cup extra-virgin olive oil
- 1 tablespoon grated orange peel (optional)

Fruit Spread

- 1 small ripe banana
- 2 cups strawberries, coarsely chopped
- 1 tablespoon orange juice

1. *To make the biscuits:* Preheat the oven to 450°F. Lightly coat a small baking sheet with cooking spray.

2. In a large bowl, whisk together the whole wheat flour, all-purpose flour, baking powder, and salt. Add the yogurt, cheese, oil, and orange peel (if using). Stir just to combine.

3. On a lightly floured surface, pat the dough into a square about 1" thick. Cut into 9 biscuits. Place on the baking sheet.

4. Bake for 10 minutes, or until the biscuits are just barely browned around the edges.

5. *To make the spread:* Meanwhile, place the banana, strawberries, and orange juice in a medium bowl. Use a potato masher or fork to mash until almost smooth. Spread on the warm biscuits.

Makes 9 servings

Per serving: 183 calories, 6 g protein, 23 g carbohydrates, 8 g total fat, 2 g saturated fat, 3 g fiber, 341 mg sodium

Fresh Berry-Oat Muffins

Prep Time: 20 minutes ★ **Total Time:** 45 minutes

For a more relaxed morning or a breakfast on the go, make these muffins the night before. If you have only one type of berry on hand, just make single-berry muffins. You can also substitute an equal amount of other chopped fresh fruit, such as peaches, apricots, apples, or pears. Freeze any remaining muffins for another meal.

1 cup old-fashioned oats

⅓ cup firmly packed light brown sugar

1 cup low-fat plain yogurt

1 egg

¾ cup whole wheat flour

½ cup oat bran

1 teaspoon baking powder

½ teaspoon baking soda

½ teaspoon salt

1 cup mixed berries, such as blueberries, blackberries, strawberries, or raspberries

1. In a large bowl, combine the oats, sugar, yogurt, and egg. Let stand for 15 minutes.

2. Meanwhile, preheat the oven to 400°F. Lightly coat 12 muffin cups with cooking spray or line with paper or foil liners.

3. In a small bowl, whisk together the flour, oat bran, baking powder, baking soda, and salt. Stir into the oat mixture just until combined. Gently fold in the berries.

4. Use a ⅓-cup measure to scoop the batter into the prepared muffin cups.

5. Bake for 15 minutes, or until the muffins are golden brown and a wooden pick inserted in the center of a muffin comes out clean. Cool in the pan on a rack for 1 minute. Remove from the pan and allow to cool for at least 10 minutes. Serve warm or at room temperature.

Makes 12 servings

Per serving: 97 calories, 4 g protein, 19 g carbohydrates, 1 g total fat, 0 g saturated fat, 2 g fiber, 220 mg sodium

Almond French Toast with Strawberries

Prep Time: 5 minutes ★ **Total Time:** 20 minutes

Serve with low-fat vanilla yogurt instead of sugary faux maple syrup.

1½ **cups sliced strawberries**

2 **teaspoons maple syrup or honey**

2 **eggs**

½ **cup 1% milk**

1 **teaspoon almond extract**

¼ **teaspoon ground cinnamon**

2 **teaspoons light olive oil**

4 **slices seven-grain or other whole grain bread**

½ **cup sliced or slivered almonds, toasted**

1. In a medium bowl, toss the strawberries and syrup or honey. Let stand for 15 minutes, tossing occasionally, or until juicy.

2. In a wide shallow bowl or pie plate, beat the eggs with a fork until blended. Add the milk, almond extract, and cinnamon and stir until blended.

3. Heat the oil in a large nonstick skillet over medium heat. Dip the bread into the egg mixture, one slice at a time, letting it sit for a few seconds to absorb the mixture. Place in the skillet and cook, turning once, for 2 minutes, or until golden. Repeat with the remaining slices.

4. Place 1 slice of bread on 4 plates. Divide the strawberries and almonds among the plates. Drizzle with any strawberry juices left in the bowl.

Makes 4 servings

Per serving: 277 calories, 11 g protein, 31 g carbohydrates, 13 g total fat, 2 g saturated fat, 5 g fiber, 239 mg sodium

Apple-Cheddar Melt

Prep Time: 10 minutes ★ **Total Time:** 15 minutes

This simple and tasty breakfast also makes a great afternoon snack.

4 slices whole grain or rye bread

4 teaspoons Dijon mustard

2 apples, cored and thinly sliced

1⅓ cups shredded reduced-fat Cheddar cheese

¼ cup finely chopped walnuts

1. Preheat the broiler. Set an oven rack 6" from the heat source. Lay the bread on a baking sheet.

2. Broil for 1½ to 2 minutes, or until just toasted. Remove the baking sheet from the oven and leave the oven on.

3. Carefully turn the bread slices. Brush each with the mustard. Top with the apples. Sprinkle evenly with the cheese and walnuts.

4. Broil for 1 to 1½ minutes, or until the cheese is melted.

5. Cut each slice in half and serve warm.

Makes 4 servings

Per serving: 255 calories, 14 g protein, 29 g carbohydrates, 12 g total fat, 5 g saturated fat, 8 g fiber, 431 mg sodium

Greek Omelets

Prep Time: 6 minutes ★ **Total Time:** 13 minutes

If you happen to have some fresh dill, add a couple of teaspoons to the beaten egg mixture. Serve with whole grain toast.

- 1 tablespoon extra-virgin olive oil, divided
- 2 packages (6 ounces each) fresh baby spinach
- 5 scallions, sliced
- 8 large eggs
- 3 tablespoons water
- ¼ teaspoon salt
- ¼ teaspoon ground black pepper
- ½ cup crumbled reduced-fat feta cheese
- 2 plum tomatoes, chopped

1. Heat 1 teaspoon of the oil in a large nonstick skillet over medium-high heat. Cook the spinach and scallions, stirring, for 1 minute, or until the spinach wilts. Remove and set aside.

2. In a large bowl, whisk the eggs, water, salt, and pepper until blended. In the same skillet, heat 1 teaspoon of the remaining oil over medium heat. Add 1 cup of the egg mixture. Cook, pushing in the edges with a spatula to let the uncooked egg flow underneath, for 2 minutes, or just until set.

3. Top half of the omelet with 1 cup of the reserved spinach mixture and sprinkle with ¼ cup of the cheese. Fold the other half over the top, reduce the heat to low, and cook for 1 minute to heat the filling and soften the cheese.

4. Using a plastic spatula, cut the omelet in half to make 2 servings. Place on 2 serving plates. Sprinkle with half of the tomato.

5. Repeat with the remaining ingredients to make 4 servings.

Makes 4 servings

Per serving: 144 calories, 13 g protein, 13 g carbohydrates, 6 g total fat, 2 g saturated fat, 5 g fiber, 630 mg sodium

Smoked Salmon and Red Onion Frittata

Prep Time: 5 minutes ★ **Total Time:** 20 minutes

Serve this open-faced baked omelet with a whole grain bagel half, toasted and brushed with olive oil, and mixed fruit or a tomato-and-olive salad on the side.

2 tablespoons extra-virgin olive oil

1 small red onion, halved and thinly sliced

6 eggs

¼ teaspoon salt

⅛ teaspoon ground black pepper

3 ounces smoked salmon

1. Preheat the oven to 400°F.

2. Heat the oil in a medium ovenproof skillet over medium heat. Cook the onion for 3 minutes, or until tender-crisp. Reduce the heat to low.

3. In a medium bowl, whisk together the eggs, salt, and pepper. Stir in the salmon. Pour over the onion. Cook for 2 to 3 minutes, or until the underside is set. Transfer the skillet to the oven.

4. Bake for 6 to 8 minutes, or until the frittata is set. Slide out onto a large round plate and cut into 4 wedges to serve.

Makes 4 servings

Per serving: 248 calories, 23 g protein, 2 g carbohydrates, 17 g total fat, 4 g saturated fat, 0 g fiber, 262 mg sodium

Italian Peppers and Eggs on Toast

Prep Time: 5 minutes ★ **Total Time:** 15 minutes

Cubanelle peppers are sometimes called Italian frying peppers. They are thin-skinned, mild, and quick cooking, so they're ideal for this recipe. Serve with sliced melon or, if in season, sliced peaches or nectarines, sprinkled with toasted sliced almonds.

1 tablespoon extra-virgin olive oil, divided

2 Cubanelle peppers, sliced

1 medium onion, thinly sliced

6 large eggs

½ teaspoon salt

⅛ teaspoon ground black pepper

4 slices whole grain Italian or French bread, toasted

¼ cup shredded reduced-fat mozzarella cheese

1. Heat 2 teaspoons of the oil in a large nonstick skillet over medium-high heat. Cook the Cubanelle peppers and onion, stirring often, for 7 minutes, or until golden and tender.

2. Meanwhile, in a medium bowl, whisk together the eggs, salt, and black pepper.

3. Reduce the heat to medium. Push the cooked peppers and onion to one side of the skillet and add the remaining 1 teaspoon oil to the other side of the skillet. Add the eggs and scramble with the peppers and onion for 1 minute, or just until the eggs are set.

4. Divide the toast, eggs, and cheese among 4 plates.

Makes 4 servings

Per serving: 240 calories, 14 g protein, 21 g carbohydrates, 12 g total fat, 3 g saturated fat, 6 g fiber, 538 mg sodium

Sun-Dried Tomato Scramble

Prep Time: 10 minutes ★ **Total Time:** 15 minutes

This is an easy yet elegant brunch dish for guests. If you have some goat cheese on hand, add an ounce or two with the tomatoes.

8 eggs

¼ cup grated Parmesan cheese

1 tablespoon finely chopped fresh basil or 1 teaspoon dried

¼ teaspoon salt

⅛ teaspoon ground black pepper

1 tablespoon extra-virgin olive oil

⅓ cup sun-dried tomatoes packed in olive oil, chopped

2 cups watercress or baby arugula

1. In a medium bowl, whisk together the eggs, cheese, basil, salt, and pepper. Heat the oil in a large nonstick skillet over medium-low heat. Cook the egg mixture for 30 seconds, or until the eggs begin to set. Add the tomatoes. Use a nonstick spoon or spatula to gently lift and mix the eggs and tomatoes together.

2. Divide the watercress or arugula and egg mixture among 4 plates.

Makes 4 servings

Per serving: 217 calories, 17 g protein, 4 g carbohydrates, 16 g total fat, 5 g saturated fat, 1 g fiber, 512 mg sodium

Warm Taco Bean Salad

Prep Time: 10 minutes ★ **Total Time:** 30 minutes

Serve with mango or pineapple chunks on the side.

1 tablespoon extra-virgin olive oil

1 onion, finely chopped

1 green bell pepper, chopped

2 cloves garlic, minced

1 teaspoon dried oregano

½ teaspoon ground cumin

½ teaspoon salt

1 can (14–19 ounces) no-salt-added kidney beans, rinsed and drained

2 tomatoes, cored and finely chopped

4 cups multigrain tortilla chips, slightly crushed

2 cups shredded romaine lettuce

1 cup shredded reduced-fat Cheddar cheese

1 avocado, chopped

½ cup green or ripe olives, sliced (optional)

¼ cup finely chopped cilantro

1. Heat the oil in a large skillet over medium heat. Cook the onion for 5 minutes, or until tender. Add the pepper, garlic, oregano, cumin, and salt. Cook, stirring, for 3 minutes, or until the pepper is tender-crisp. Remove from the heat and stir in the beans and tomatoes.

2. Divide the chips, lettuce, bean mixture, cheese, avocado, olives (if using), and cilantro among 4 plates.

Makes 4 servings

Per serving: 379 calories, 16 g protein, 42 g carbohydrates, 19 g total fat, 4 g saturated fat, 12 g fiber, 588 mg sodium

Warm Chicken Salad

Prep Time: 10 minutes ★ **Total Time:** 35 minutes

On the side, serve crusty whole grain rolls with a little extra-virgin olive oil in individual saucers for dipping.

1 pound boneless, skinless chicken breast halves

1 tablespoon sliced garlic

½ teaspoon salt, divided

2 red bell peppers

6 cups baby arugula or spinach leaves

¼ cup extra-virgin olive oil

2 tablespoons balsamic vinegar or lemon juice

⅛ teaspoon ground black pepper

¼ cup pine nuts, toasted

1. In a large saucepan, combine the chicken, garlic, and ¼ teaspoon of the salt with enough water to cover by 1". Bring to a boil over high heat. Reduce the heat to medium-low and simmer for 20 minutes, or until the chicken is just cooked through. Drain off the water and set the chicken aside to cool slightly.

2. Meanwhile, preheat the broiler. Place the bell peppers on a broiler pan. Broil 2" from the heat source, turning often, for 15 minutes, or until blackened all over. Set aside until cool enough to handle.

3. Shred the reserved chicken and place in a large bowl. Remove and discard the core and seeds from the reserved peppers. Cut into thin slices and add to the bowl. Add the arugula or spinach, oil, vinegar or lemon juice, black pepper, and the remaining ¼ teaspoon salt. Toss gently to mix.

4. Divide among 4 plates. Sprinkle with the pine nuts.

Makes 4 servings

Per serving: 349 calories, 27 g protein, 8 g carbohydrates, 23 g total fat, 3 g saturated fat, 2 g fiber, 435 mg sodium

Couscous Salad with Shrimp and Lemon-Dill Dressing

Prep Time: 10 minutes ★ **Total Time:** 40 minutes

Whole wheat couscous is a fast way to get whole grains into your diet. This main-dish salad keeps well, so it can be prepared up to 2 days ahead. Serve with low-fat, reduced-sodium tomato soup.

1 cup whole wheat couscous

1 teaspoon + 3 tablespoons extra-virgin olive oil

½ teaspoon salt, divided

1 medium tomato, chopped

½ medium cucumber, seeded and chopped

3 scallions, sliced

¼ cup chopped dill

1 teaspoon freshly grated lemon peel

3 tablespoons lemon juice

¼ teaspoon ground black pepper

½ pound cooked, peeled, and deveined large shrimp, halved crosswise

⅓ cup crumbled reduced-fat feta cheese

1. Prepare the couscous according to package directions, adding 1 teaspoon of the oil and ¼ teaspoon of the salt. Fluff with a fork and set aside for 20 minutes, or until at room temperature.

2. Meanwhile, in a large bowl, combine the tomato, cucumber, scallions, dill, lemon peel, lemon juice, pepper, 3 tablespoons of the oil, and the remaining ¼ teaspoon salt. Toss to mix. Set aside, tossing occasionally, for 15 minutes, or until the tomato releases its juice.

3. Add the reserved couscous, shrimp, and cheese. Toss to coat well.

Makes 4 servings

Per serving: 302 calories, 18 g protein, 28 g carbohydrates, 14 g total fat, 3 g saturated fat, 5 g fiber, 272 mg sodium

Cold Asian Noodle Salad

Prep Time: 20 minutes ★ **Total Time:** 25 minutes

These noodles don't have to be ice-cold—you can serve them at room temperature as well as straight from the refrigerator. If you like, you can add other vegetables, such as sliced snow peas, cut-up green beans, slivered radishes, or halved cherry tomatoes. Otherwise, serve those vegetables with shredded lettuce as part of a crisp side salad.

1 tablespoon light olive oil

1 tablespoon finely chopped fresh ginger

2 cloves garlic, minced

¼ cup peanut butter

2 tablespoons light soy sauce

2 tablespoons Asian sesame oil

2 tablespoons lemon juice

8 ounces angel hair pasta or soba (buckwheat) noodles

2 scallions, thinly sliced

1 large carrot, shredded

1. Heat the olive oil in a small saucepan over medium heat. Cook the ginger and garlic for 30 seconds. Stir in the peanut butter, soy sauce, sesame oil, and lemon juice. Cook, stirring often, for 2 minutes. Set aside.

2. Prepare the pasta or noodles according to package directions. Rinse under cold running water. Drain well.

3. In a large bowl, toss together the noodles, scallions, and carrot. Add the reserved dressing and toss to coat.

NOTE: If the dressing gets too thick while standing, thin with a spoonful or two of boiling water.

Makes 4 servings

Per serving: 413 calories, 12 g protein, 48 g carbohydrates, 20 g total fat, 3 g saturated fat, 3 g fiber, 390 mg sodium

Tabbouleh with Chickpeas and Artichoke Hearts

Prep Time: 1 hour 10 minutes ★ **Total Time:** 1 hour 10 minutes

Prepare the vegetables and seasonings while the bulgur is soaking. You can also make this hearty grain salad with quinoa or whole wheat couscous. If you do, skip step 1 and instead follow the package directions for cooking these grains before adding the other ingredients.

1½ cups water

1 cup fine bulgur

2 cups finely chopped parsley

2 large tomatoes, cored and finely chopped

1 cucumber, peeled, seeded, and chopped

1 can (15 ounces) no-salt-added chickpeas, rinsed and drained

1 jar (6 ounces) artichoke hearts, drained and finely chopped

5 scallions, thinly sliced, or 1 small red onion, finely chopped

⅓ cup olive oil

⅓ cup lemon juice

¼ cup finely chopped fresh mint or 1 tablespoon dried

1 teaspoon salt

¼ teaspoon ground black pepper

Romaine lettuce leaves and hearts

1. Bring the water to a boil. In a large bowl, stir together the bulgur and water. Cover and let stand at room temperature for 1 hour.

2. Add the parsley, tomatoes, cucumber, chickpeas, artichoke hearts, scallions or onion, oil, lemon juice, mint, salt, and pepper.

3. Divide among 8 plates. Use the lettuce to scoop up the tabbouleh.

Makes 8 servings

Per serving: 233 calories, 5 g protein, 26 g carbohydrates, 13 g total fat, 2 g saturated fat, 6 g fiber, 379 mg sodium

Caponata

Prep Time: 15 minutes ★ **Total Time:** 1 hour 10 minutes + marinating time

This classic Italian make-ahead, sweet-and-sour vegetable combination can be served with feta cheese and whole wheat pitas for lunch, spread on toasted slices of whole grain baguette for a snack, or presented as a vegetable side dish with dinner.

½ cup extra-virgin olive oil, divided

2 medium eggplants, cut into ½" cubes (2 pounds)

4 ribs celery, peeled and coarsely chopped

1 onion, finely chopped

2 large tomatoes, cored, seeded, and coarsely chopped

½ cup fresh basil, chopped, or 1 tablespoon dried, divided

2 anchovies, chopped

1 cup pitted green or ripe olives or a mixture, coarsely chopped

¼ cup pine nuts (optional)

¼ cup raisins

⅓ cup balsamic vinegar

2 tablespoons drained capers

½ teaspoon salt

1. Heat ¼ cup of the oil in a large skillet over medium heat. Cook the eggplant for 10 minutes, stirring occasionally. Transfer to a bowl and set aside.

2. Heat the remaining ¼ cup oil in the same skillet. Cook the celery and onion for 5 minutes, or until tender. Stir in the tomatoes, half of the basil, the anchovies, olives, pine nuts (if using), raisins, vinegar, capers, and salt. Cook for 30 minutes, stirring occasionally.

3. Stir in the reserved eggplant and cook for 10 minutes.

4. Transfer to a serving bowl or storage container. Stir in the remaining basil. Cover and refrigerate for at least 8 hours or up to 3 days. Serve at room temperature.

Makes 6 servings

Per serving: 279 calories, 3 g protein, 21 g carbohydrates, 22 g total fat, 3 g saturated fat, 7 g fiber, 490 mg sodium

Roasted Beet, Apple, and Walnut Salad

Prep Time: 15 minutes ★ **Total Time:** 45 minutes

In a pinch, you can simply boil the beets or use drained, canned beets in place of fresh.

4 **beets, peeled and quartered**

¼ **cup extra-virgin olive oil, divided**

2 **tablespoons orange juice**

1 **tablespoon balsamic vinegar**

⅛ **teaspoon salt**

⅛ **teaspoon ground black pepper**

2 **apples, chopped**

1 **rib celery, peeled and thinly sliced**

½ **cup walnuts, finely chopped**

4 **cups baby spinach or mixed baby greens**

1. Preheat the oven to 425°F. Divide the beets between two 12" sheets of foil. Drizzle each with 1 tablespoon of the oil. Loosely wrap the beets in the foil and place on a baking sheet.

2. Roast for 25 minutes, or until the beets are just tender when pierced with a fork. Open the foil packets to allow the beets to cool.

3. Meanwhile, in a medium bowl, whisk together the orange juice, vinegar, salt, pepper, and the remaining 2 tablespoons oil. Add the apples, celery, and walnuts and toss gently to coat. Add the beets to the bowl.

4. Divide the spinach or baby greens and the salad among 4 plates.

Makes 4 servings

Per serving: 316 calories, 4 g protein, 25 g carbohydrates, 24 g total fat, 3 g saturated fat, 7 g fiber, 199 mg sodium

Pasta Salad with Tuna, Eggs, and Red Beans

Prep Time: 25 minutes ★ **Total Time:** 25 minutes

You can make this salad with leftover fresh tuna, if you happen to have any on hand.

8 ounces whole grain penne, rotelle, or other stubby pasta shape

¼ cup extra-virgin olive oil

2 tablespoons lemon juice

1 tablespoon mayonnaise

½ teaspoon salt

2 cans (5 ounces each) light or white albacore tuna packed in water, drained

2 hard-cooked eggs, quartered

1 cup cherry tomatoes, halved

1 cup canned red kidney beans, rinsed and drained

1. Prepare the pasta according to package directions. Rinse under cold water and drain completely.

2. In a large bowl, whisk together the oil, lemon juice, mayonnaise, and salt. Add the pasta and toss to coat.

3. Add the tuna, eggs, tomatoes, and beans. Gently toss just to combine.

Makes 4 servings

Per serving: 415 calories, 25 g protein, 19 g carbohydrates, 4 g total fat, 4 g saturated fat, 5 g fiber, 683 mg sodium

Turkey Salad Plate

Prep Time: 20 minutes ★ **Total Time:** 25 minutes

Roast a turkey breast on Sunday so you have leftovers to use during the week for salads and sandwiches.

- 1 **pound green beans**
- 2 **tablespoons extra-virgin olive oil**
- 2 **tablespoons lemon juice**
- ½ **teaspoon dried thyme, crushed**
- ¼ **teaspoon salt**
- 2 **scallions, thinly sliced**

- 1 **tomato, cored and chopped**
- 1 **tablespoon mayonnaise**
- 12 **ounces roast turkey breast, chopped**
- 1 **large rib celery, peeled and thinly sliced**
- ⅓ **cup pitted ripe olives, sliced**

1. Place a steamer basket in a large pot with 2" of water over medium-high heat. Steam the green beans for 5 minutes, or until tender-crisp. Drain and set aside.

2. Meanwhile, in a medium bowl, whisk together the oil, lemon juice, thyme, and salt. Transfer 2 tablespoons of the dressing to another medium bowl and set aside.

3. Add the scallions, tomato, and reserved green beans to the first bowl. Toss to mix well.

4. Whisk the mayonnaise into the reserved dressing in the second bowl. Add the turkey, celery, and olives. Toss to mix well.

5. Divide the turkey salad and green bean salad evenly among 4 plates.

Makes 4 servings

Per serving: 261 calories, 28 g protein, 11 g carbohydrates, 12 g total fat, 2 g saturated fat, 4 g fiber, 291 mg sodium

Shrimp and Avocado Salad
with Lime Vinaigrette

Prep Time: 20 minutes ★ **Total Time:** 30 minutes

To save time and avoid cooking, use 12 ounces of precooked, shelled shrimp. In that case, eliminate 1 tablespoon of the olive oil, and rub the garlic on the inside of the mixing bowl before you add the other ingredients. Serve with sliced watermelon on the side.

3 **tablespoons extra-virgin olive oil, divided**

1 **pound shrimp, shelled and deveined**

2 **cloves garlic, minced**

2 **tablespoons lime juice**

¼ **teaspoon salt**

1 **cup cherry tomatoes, halved**

1 **avocado, halved, pitted, peeled, and sliced**

1 **small red onion, halved and thinly sliced**

¼ **cup finely chopped cilantro**

4 **cups fresh baby spinach or arugula**

1. Heat 1 tablespoon of the oil in a large skillet over medium-high heat. Cook the shrimp and garlic, stirring often, for 4 minutes, or until opaque. Set aside to cool.

2. In a large bowl, whisk together the lime juice, salt, and the remaining 2 tablespoons oil. Add the tomatoes, avocado, onion, cilantro, and the reserved shrimp. Toss gently.

3. Divide the greens and salad among 4 plates.

Makes 4 servings

Per serving: 285 calories, 22 g protein, 11 g carbohydrates, 18 g total fat, 2.5 g saturated fat, 4 g fiber, 337 mg sodium

Pita Pizzas

Prep Time: 10 minutes ★ **Total Time:** 20 minutes

Serve these simple pies with a crisp green salad tossed with olive oil vinaigrette.

4 low-carbohydrate or high-fiber pitas (6")

1½ cups shredded reduced-fat four-cheese Italian-style blend, divided

3 tomatoes, thinly sliced

1 teaspoon dried oregano, crumbled

⅓ cup pitted kalamata or other ripe olives, thinly sliced

2 tablespoons pine nuts

1. Move the oven rack to the bottom third of the oven. Preheat the oven to 400°F.

2. Place the pitas on a baking sheet. Sprinkle evenly with 1 cup of the cheese. Top with the tomatoes, oregano, olives, pine nuts, and the remaining ½ cup cheese.

3. Bake for 8 minutes, or until the cheese is melted and the pitas are crisp around the edges.

Makes 4 servings

Per serving: 211 calories, 16 g protein, 12 g carbohydrates, 12 g total fat, 5 g saturated fat, 4 g fiber, 516 mg sodium

English Muffin Pizzas

Prep Time: 15 minutes ★ **Total Time:** 25 minutes

This mixture is also great spread on whole grain crackers or pita wedges for a snack. Although freshly roasted peppers are used in this recipe, to save time, substitute 1 cup bottled roasted peppers instead. Serve with an arugula, grape tomato, and red onion salad.

4 **whole grain English muffins, split and toasted**

1 **can (14–19 ounces) cannellini beans, rinsed and drained**

1 **tablespoon extra-virgin olive oil**

1 **teaspoon minced garlic**

¼ **teaspoon salt**

2 **whole roasted red peppers, cut into strips**

½ **cup shredded reduced-fat mozzarella cheese**

4 **teaspoons grated Parmesan cheese**

1. Preheat the oven to 425°F. Place the muffins on a baking sheet.

2. In a medium bowl, combine the beans, oil, garlic, and salt. Mash with a potato masher or fork until spreadable.

3. Spread about 2 tablespoons onto each muffin half. Divide the peppers evenly over each. Top each with 1 tablespoon of the mozzarella and ½ teaspoon of the Parmesan.

4. Bake for 8 minutes, or until the cheese is melted.

Makes 4 servings

Per serving: 296 calories, 14 g protein, 43 g carbohydrates, 8 g total fat, 2 g saturated fat, 5 g fiber, 756 mg sodium

Tuna Salad Sandwich

Prep Time: 10 minutes ★ **Total Time:** 10 minutes

This is a great make-ahead sandwich because the flavor gets better after it sits awhile. Serve with baked vegetable chips, pickles, or cucumber spears.

3 tablespoons extra-virgin olive oil

3 tablespoons red wine vinegar

2 tablespoons chopped fresh oregano or ½ teaspoon dried

1 teaspoon minced garlic

4 crusty whole grain rolls (5"–6" long), split

4 cups baby arugula

2 cans (5 ounces each) water-packed chunk white albacore tuna, drained

1 jar (7 ounces) roasted peppers, drained and cut into strips

1 small onion, thinly sliced

¼ cup sliced pitted kalamata olives

1. In a small bowl, whisk the oil, vinegar, oregano, and garlic until blended. Pull out about ½ cup bread from the inside of each roll. (Save to make bread crumbs.)

2. Drizzle 1 tablespoon of the oil mixture over the cut surfaces of each roll. Top the bottom half of each roll with 1 cup of the arugula.

3. In a medium bowl, combine the tuna, peppers, onion, and olives. Add the remaining oil mixture and toss to coat. Place ¾ cup of the tuna mixture on top of the arugula. Top with the roll tops.

4. If not serving immediately, wrap each sandwich tightly in plastic wrap. Set aside at room temperature for 1 hour or refrigerate for up to 1 day for the flavors to blend and intensify.

Makes 4 servings

Per serving: 264 calories, 17 g protein, 17 g carbohydrates, 14 g total fat, 2 g saturated fat, 3 g fiber, 513 mg sodium

Turkey–Black Bean Burgers

Prep Time: 10 minutes ★ **Total Time:** 20 minutes

We reduced the amount of meat in these flavorful burgers by adding beans and vegetables. Serve with a few baked tortilla chips and a sliced cucumber and red onion salad tossed with olive oil, lime juice, and cilantro.

1 cup canned black beans, rinsed and drained

1 egg white

2 medium carrots, shredded

4 scallions, sliced

½ cup chopped cilantro, divided

1½ teaspoons ground cumin

¼ teaspoon salt

½ pound lean ground turkey

1½ tablespoons extra-virgin olive oil

¾ cup salsa

2 cups shredded romaine lettuce

1. Put the beans in a large bowl and coarsely mash with a potato masher. Add the egg white, carrots, scallions, ¼ cup of the cilantro, cumin, and salt and mix until combined. Add the turkey and mix well. Shape into 4 (½"-thick) burgers.

2. Heat the oil in a large nonstick skillet over medium heat. Cook the burgers, turning once, for 8 to 10 minutes, or until a thermometer inserted in the centers registers 165°F and the meat is no longer pink.

3. In a small bowl, stir together the salsa and the remaining ¼ cup cilantro. For each serving, place ½ cup of the lettuce on a plate, then top with a burger and 3 tablespoons of the salsa mixture.

Makes 4 servings

Per serving: 311 calories, 47 g protein, 18 g carbohydrates, 8 g total fat, 1 g saturated fat, 6 g fiber, 859 mg sodium

Crustless Zucchini Quiche

Prep Time: 15 minutes ★ **Total Time:** 55 minutes

If you're serving salad, place a slice of quiche right on top of the dressed greens for a more sophisticated presentation. A bowl of bean or lentil soup on the side will round out the meal.

1 tablespoon olive oil

1 onion, chopped

2 zucchini, halved lengthwise and thinly sliced

1 teaspoon dried rosemary, crushed

3 eggs

½ cup milk

1 teaspoon Dijon mustard

½ teaspoon salt

2 cups shredded reduced-fat four-cheese Italian-style blend

2 tablespoons pine nuts

1. Preheat the oven to 350°F. Coat a 9" pie plate with cooking spray.

2. Heat the oil in a large skillet over medium heat. Cook the onion, zucchini, and rosemary, stirring often, for 10 minutes, or until tender.

3. Meanwhile, in a large bowl, whisk together the eggs, milk, mustard, and salt. Stir in the cheese.

4. Spoon the zucchini mixture into the pie plate. Top with the egg mixture. Sprinkle with the pine nuts.

5. Bake for 20 to 25 minutes, or until a knife inserted into the center of the quiche comes out clean. Cool on a rack for 10 minutes.

Makes 6 servings

Per serving: 216 calories, 16 g protein, 7 g carbohydrates, 13 g total fat, 5.5 g saturated fat, 1 g fiber, 557 mg sodium

Tomato Lentil Soup

Prep Time: 15 minutes ★ **Total Time:** 50 minutes

Serve this soup with a crisp green salad topped with crumbled goat or feta cheese and a toasted slice of whole grain pita.

2 tablespoons extra-virgin olive oil

1 onion, finely chopped

1 large carrot, chopped

1 rib celery, chopped

1 tablespoon minced garlic

1 tablespoon minced fresh ginger

1 tablespoon curry powder

1½ cups lentils, picked over and rinsed

2 cans (14½ ounces each) low-fat, reduced-sodium chicken or vegetable broth, or water

4 large tomatoes, seeded and chopped, or 1 can (28 ounces) diced tomatoes in juice

½ teaspoon salt

½ cup finely chopped cilantro

1. Heat the oil in a large saucepan over medium heat. Cook the onion, carrot, celery, garlic, ginger, and curry powder for 5 minutes, or until tender.

2. Add the lentils and broth or water. Heat to a boil over medium-high heat. Reduce the heat to low, cover, and simmer, stirring occasionally, for 20 minutes, or until the lentils are just tender. Add a little more water, if necessary, to keep the lentils covered in liquid.

3. Stir in the tomatoes and salt. Simmer for 10 minutes. Stir in the cilantro just before serving.

Makes 8 servings

Per serving: 176 calories, 9 g protein, 27 g carbohydrates, 5 g total fat, 0.5 g saturated fat, 7 g fiber, 394 mg sodium

Root Vegetable Soup

Prep Time: 15 minutes ★ **Total Time:** 1 hour 5 minutes

You can experiment with using parsnips, kohlrabi, and celery root in place of some of the carrots and potatoes. If you're feeling really ambitious, you can cut the vegetables into larger chunks, toss in olive oil, and roast in a preheated 400°F oven for 30 to 45 minutes before adding to the soup. Serve with bean salad for a balanced meal.

2 tablespoons olive oil

1 onion, chopped

2 cloves garlic, minced

3 carrots, chopped

2 ribs celery, chopped

2 small new potatoes, peeled and chopped

1 turnip, chopped

1 can (14½ ounces) low-fat, reduced-sodium chicken or vegetable broth

½ cup low-fat evaporated milk

1 bay leaf

½ teaspoon salt

¼ teaspoon dried thyme

2 cups shredded reduced-fat Cheddar cheese

1. Heat the oil in a large saucepan over medium heat. Cook the onion for 5 minutes, or until tender. Add the garlic and cook for 1 minute.

2. Add the carrots, celery, potatoes, turnip, broth, milk, bay leaf, salt, and thyme. Heat to a boil over medium-high heat. Reduce the heat to medium-low, cover, and simmer for 40 minutes, or until the vegetables are very tender. Remove the bay leaf from the soup.

3. Use a potato masher or fork to mash some of the vegetables to thicken the soup.

4. Remove from the heat and gradually stir in the cheese until melted.

Makes 4 servings

Per serving: 282 calories, 20 g protein, 16 g carbohydrates, 17 g total fat, 7.5 g saturated fat, 3 g fiber, 855 mg sodium

Minestrone Soup with Barley

Prep Time: 10 minutes ★ **Total Time:** 45 minutes

This classic Italian soup is usually made with pasta. We used barley instead, which is full of fiber, vitamins, and minerals and may help stabilize glucose levels. Serve with whole grain crackers or breadsticks.

1 tablespoon extra-virgin olive oil

1 onion, chopped

1½ tablespoons minced garlic

1¾ cups water

1 can (14½ ounces) low-fat, reduced-sodium chicken or vegetable broth

½ cup barley

1 can (14½ ounces) diced tomatoes in juice

2 small zucchini, chopped

¼ pound green beans, cut into 1½" pieces

1 medium carrot, chopped

3 tablespoons grated Parmesan cheese

1. Heat the oil in a large saucepan over medium-high heat. Cook the onion, stirring, for 5 minutes, or until lightly browned. Add the garlic and cook for 1 minute.

2. Stir in the water, broth, and barley and bring to a boil over medium-high heat. Reduce the heat to medium-low, cover, and simmer, stirring occasionally, for 20 minutes, or until the barley is almost tender.

3. Add the tomatoes, zucchini, green beans, and carrot and bring to a boil over medium-high heat. Reduce the heat to medium-low, cover, and simmer, stirring occasionally, for 10 minutes, or until the barley and vegetables are tender.

4. Remove from the heat and stir in the cheese.

Makes 4 servings

Per serving: 202 calories, 7 g protein, 33 g carbohydrates, 5 g total fat, 1 g saturated fat, 7 g fiber, 474 mg sodium

Poblano Chile and Bean Soup

Prep Time: 10 minutes ★ **Total Time:** 25 minutes

Poblano peppers are mild as far as chile peppers go, but they still pack a bit of heat. If you don't like spicy food, use a bell or Cubanelle pepper instead. Serve with a sliced avocado and orange salad, sprinkled with toasted pumpkin seeds.

2 teaspoons extra-virgin olive oil

1 onion, chopped

1 poblano chile pepper, chopped (wear plastic gloves when handling)

½ cup fresh or frozen and thawed corn kernels

2 teaspoons minced garlic

1 can (14½ ounces) low-fat, reduced-sodium chicken or vegetable broth

½ teaspoon chili powder

½ teaspoon ground cumin

1 can (14–19 ounces) pinto beans, rinsed and drained

⅓ cup chopped cilantro

1½ tablespoons lime juice

1. Heat the oil in a medium saucepan over medium-high heat. Cook the onion, pepper, and corn, stirring occasionally, for 8 minutes, or until the vegetables are light golden. Add the garlic and cook over low heat for 1 minute, or until fragrant.

2. Stir in the broth, chili powder, and cumin and bring to a boil over medium-high heat. Reduce the heat to low, stir in the beans, and cook for 5 minutes for the flavors to blend.

3. Remove from the heat and stir in the cilantro and lime juice.

Makes 4 servings

Per serving: 118 calories, 5 g protein, 17 g carbohydrates, 3 g total fat, 0.5 g saturated fat, 5 g fiber, 351 mg sodium

Gazpacho with Avocado

Prep Time: 20 minutes ★ **Total Time:** 20 minutes + chilling time

This chunky, refreshing vegetable soup is the perfect starter or side dish on a hot day when you don't feel like turning on the stove. Serve with cold sliced chicken or turkey or shrimp and a slice of whole grain baguette, toasted and brushed with olive oil—or with a sandwich made with reduced-fat cheese on whole grain bread.

4 scallions, coarsely chopped

3 tomatoes, coarsely chopped

2 large cloves garlic

2 ribs celery, coarsely chopped

1 yellow or orange bell pepper, coarsely chopped

1 English cucumber, coarsely chopped

2 cups low-sodium tomato or vegetable juice

2 tablespoons extra-virgin olive oil

2 tablespoons balsamic vinegar

½ teaspoon sea salt

Pinch of red-pepper flakes (optional)

1 avocado, chopped

1. In a food processor, finely chop the scallions, tomatoes, and garlic. Spoon into a large bowl or pitcher. Repeat with the celery, bell pepper, and cucumber.

2. Stir in the juice, oil, vinegar, salt, and pepper flakes (if using). Refrigerate for at least 4 hours or up to 2 days before serving.

3. Spoon the cold soup into 8 bowls. Sprinkle each serving with 2 tablespoons of the avocado.

Makes 8 servings

Per serving: 97 calories, 2 g protein, 9 g carbohydrates, 6 g total fat, 1 g saturated fat, 3 g fiber, 136 mg sodium

Nut-Crusted Chicken Fingers

Prep Time: 20 minutes ★ **Total Time:** 40 minutes

You can use chopped walnuts, hazelnuts, or even peanuts in place of the almonds, if you like.

1 **cup sliced natural almonds**

2 **teaspoons paprika**

¼ **teaspoon salt**

½ **cup low-fat plain yogurt**

1 **egg white**

¼ **cup grated Parmesan cheese**

1 **pound chicken tenders**

1. Preheat the oven to 425°F. Lightly coat a large baking sheet with cooking spray.

2. In a food processor, combine the almonds, paprika, and salt. Process until the almonds are finely ground. Transfer to a plate.

3. In a wide shallow dish or pie plate, whisk together the yogurt, egg white, and cheese. Dip the chicken in the yogurt mixture, then in the almonds to coat. Place on the prepared baking sheet.

4. Bake for 15 to 20 minutes, or until the coating is crisp and the chicken is no longer pink in the center and the juices run clear.

Makes 4 servings

Per serving: 282 calories, 35 g protein, 8 g carbohydrates, 14 g total fat, 2 g saturated fat, 3 g fiber, 299 mg sodium

Grilled Chicken Milanese

Prep Time: 20 minutes ★ **Total Time:** 25 minutes

Chicken Milanese is typically breaded and fried. Here it is prepared much more healthfully by grilling. Add 1 cup rinsed and drained canned cannellini beans to the arugula topping, if desired. If you don't add the beans, serve with whole grain bread, toasted and brushed with olive oil.

¼ cup extra-virgin olive oil

2 tablespoons red wine vinegar

1 clove garlic, minced

½ teaspoon dried oregano

¼ teaspoon salt

¼ teaspoon ground black pepper

4 chicken breast cutlets (about 4 ounces each)

4 cups baby arugula

1 large tomato, chopped

½ small red onion, thinly sliced

1. In a shallow bowl large enough to hold the chicken, combine the oil, vinegar, garlic, oregano, salt, and pepper. Remove half the mixture, place in a large bowl, and set aside.

2. Add the chicken to the shallow bowl and marinate for 15 minutes. Remove the chicken from the marinade. Discard the marinade.

3. Coat a grill rack or grill pan with cooking spray and preheat.

4. Place the chicken on the grill rack or grill pan. Cook, turning once, for 4 minutes, or until no longer pink and the juices run clear.

5. Meanwhile, add the arugula, tomato, and onion to the bowl with the reserved dressing. Toss to coat well. Divide among 4 plates. Top each with a chicken cutlet.

Makes 4 servings

Per serving: 275 calories, 25 g protein, 4 g carbohydrates, 17 g total fat, 3 g saturated fat, 1 g fiber, 286 mg sodium

Garlic-Herb Roasted Chicken and Vegetables

Prep Time: 10 minutes ★ **Total Time:** 50 minutes

This one-dish meal is easy on the cleanup. Any leftovers will make a great lunch the next day.

1 whole chicken (about 4 pounds), cut-up and skinned

1 large head cauliflower, cut in florets

8 carrots, cut in 3" pieces

8 small red potatoes, halved

1 bulb garlic, separated into cloves, unpeeled

¼ cup extra-virgin olive oil, divided

2 tablespoons chopped fresh oregano or 1 teaspoon dried, divided

1 tablespoon chopped fresh thyme or ½ teaspoon dried, divided

½ teaspoon salt, divided

8 pitted kalamata olives, chopped

Balsamic vinegar

1. Preheat the oven to 425°F. Divide the chicken, cauliflower, carrots, potatoes, and garlic between 2 large rimmed baking sheets. Drizzle each pan with 2 tablespoons of the oil. Sprinkle each with half of the oregano, thyme, and salt. Toss to coat.

2. Roast for 25 minutes. Remove the pans from the oven. Toss the vegetables and turn the chicken. Return to the oven and roast for 15 minutes, or until a thermometer inserted in the thickest portion of the chicken registers 170°F, the juices run clear, and the vegetables are tender.

3. Place the chicken and vegetables on a serving platter. Squeeze the roasted garlic over the chicken and vegetables and toss to coat. Sprinkle with the olives and pass the vinegar at the table.

Makes 8 servings

Per serving: 384 calories, 29 g protein, 41 g carbohydrates, 12 g total fat, 2 g saturated fat, 7 g fiber, 373 mg sodium

Brown Rice–Stuffed Peppers

Prep Time: 25 minutes ★ **Total Time:** 1 hour 15 minutes

You can substitute an equal amount of prepared whole wheat couscous for the rice.

2 large red, yellow, or orange bell peppers, halved lengthwise, cored, and seeded

2 tablespoons extra-virgin olive oil

1 onion, chopped

⅓ cup walnuts, chopped

2 cloves garlic, minced

1 cup cooked brown rice

⅓ cup raisins

½ teaspoon salt

⅛ teaspoon ground black pepper

4 ounces goat cheese, crumbled

1 tablespoon chopped fresh parsley

1. Preheat the oven to 400°F. Place the bell pepper halves in a large baking pan.

2. Heat the oil in a large skillet over medium heat. Cook the onion for 5 minutes, or until lightly browned. Add the walnuts and cook, stirring occasionally, for 5 minutes. Add the garlic and cook for 1 minute.

3. Stir in the rice, raisins, salt, and black pepper. Cook for 5 minutes. Remove the skillet from the heat and stir in the goat cheese and parsley. Divide the mixture among the bell pepper halves.

4. Bake for 35 minutes, or until the bell peppers are tender.

Makes 4 servings

Per serving: 364 calories, 10 g protein, 31 g carbohydrates, 23 g total fat, 7.5 g saturated fat, 5 g fiber, 448 mg sodium

Linguine "Bolognese"

Prep Time: 10 minutes ★ **Total Time:** 25 minutes

Meaty mushrooms stand in for beef in this lusty sauce. If you prefer, chop the vegetables in a food processor.

8 ounces whole wheat linguine or spaghetti

2½ tablespoons olive oil

1 onion, chopped

1 medium carrot, chopped

8 ounces baby bella or other mushrooms, chopped

2½ teaspoons minced garlic

½ cup dry red wine

1½ cups canned crushed tomatoes

½ teaspoon dried rosemary

⅛ teaspoon red-pepper flakes

¼ cup grated Parmesan cheese

1. Prepare the pasta according to package directions, reserving ½ cup of the cooking water before draining.

2. Meanwhile, heat the oil in a large skillet over medium-high heat. Cook the onion and carrot for 5 minutes, or until the onion is lightly browned.

3. Add the mushrooms and garlic and cook, stirring, for 3 minutes, or until the mushrooms are softened.

4. Stir in the wine and cook for 1 minute. Add the tomatoes, rosemary, and pepper flakes and bring to a boil over medium-high heat. Reduce the heat to low and simmer, stirring occasionally, for 5 minutes.

5. Add the pasta and reserved cooking water to the skillet and toss to coat. Divide among 4 bowls and sprinkle with the cheese.

Makes 4 servings

Per serving: 393 calories, 14 g protein, 58 g carbohydrates, 11 g total fat, 2 g saturated fat, 10 g fiber, 223 mg sodium

Noodle-Free Eggplant Lasagna

Prep Time: 30 minutes ★ **Total Time:** 1 hour 15 minutes

This dish has all the makings of a classic vegetarian lasagna, without the extra carbs. That means you can enjoy a slice or two of whole grain garlic bread on the side.

1 large eggplant, peeled and sliced into 18 rounds (¼" thick), salted, and drained

1 tablespoon + ½ teaspoon salt

2 tablespoons extra-virgin olive oil

1 onion, finely chopped

2 cloves garlic, minced

1 red bell pepper, finely chopped

4 cups fresh baby spinach

2 cups no-salt-added tomato sauce, divided

2 eggs

2 cups part-skim ricotta cheese

1 cup shredded reduced-fat four-cheese Italian-style blend

⅓ cup grated Parmesan cheese

1. Preheat the oven to 425°F. Lightly coat a 13" × 9" baking dish with cooking spray.

2. To remove any bitterness from the eggplant before using it, place the slices in a large colander and toss with 1 tablespoon of the salt. Let stand for 15 minutes, or until moisture is released from the eggplant. Rinse the eggplant with running water and pat dry with a paper towel.

3. Meanwhile, heat the oil in a large saucepan over medium heat. Cook the onion for 5 minutes, or until lightly browned. Add the garlic and cook for 1 minute. Add the bell pepper, spinach, and ½ teaspoon salt. Cook, stirring occasionally, for 5 minutes. Stir in 1 cup of the tomato sauce.

4. In a medium bowl, stir together the eggs, ricotta, and cheese blend until well mixed.

5. Spread the remaining 1 cup tomato sauce in the bottom of the baking dish. Arrange the 6 largest eggplant slices in a single layer over the sauce. Top each slice with ¼ cup of the vegetable mixture. Top each with a spoonful of the cheese mixture and another eggplant slice. Repeat the layering, ending with the cheese mixture. Sprinkle the Parmesan evenly over the eggplant stacks. Cover loosely with foil.

6. Bake for 30 to 45 minutes, or until the mixture is bubbly and the eggplant is very tender. Cool on a rack for 10 minutes before serving.

Makes 6 servings

Per serving: 333 calories, 23 g protein, 22 g carbohydrates, 18 g total fat, 8 g saturated fat, 7 g fiber, 811 mg sodium

Grilled Portobello Burgers

Prep Time: 10 minutes ★ **Total Time:** 25 minutes

For cheeseburgers, after grilling the mushrooms, fill each cap with 2 tablespoons shredded reduced-fat mozzarella cheese and grill about 1 minute, or until the cheese melts. Serve with a salad of shredded carrots, sliced scallions, and chopped parsley dressed with olive oil and red wine vinegar and sprinkled with chopped toasted almonds.

Aioli

- 3 tablespoons reduced-fat mayonnaise
- 2 tablespoons chopped fresh basil
- ½ teaspoon minced garlic
- ½ teaspoon red wine vinegar

Burgers

- 2 tablespoons extra-virgin olive oil
- ¼ teaspoon salt
- ¼ teaspoon ground black pepper
- 4 large portobello mushroom caps
- 1 large sweet onion, cut into 4 thick slices
- 4 whole grain hamburger rolls
- 8 large leaves basil
- 2 tomatoes, each cut into 4 thick slices

1. Coat a grill rack or a broiler pan with cooking spray. Preheat the grill or broiler.

2. *To make the aioli:* In a small cup, stir together the mayonnaise, basil, garlic, and vinegar until combined. Set aside.

3. *To make the burgers:* In a small cup, combine the oil, salt, and pepper. Brush the mushrooms and onion slices with the oil mixture and place on the grill rack or broiler pan. Grill or broil, turning once, for 10 minutes, or until lightly charred and tender. Remove to a platter.

4. Place the rolls, cut side down, on the grill rack or broiler pan and cook for 1 minute, or until lightly toasted.

5. Spread the bottoms of the rolls with the aioli. Top each with 2 basil leaves, 2 tomato slices, an onion slice, a mushroom, and the top of the roll.

Makes 4 servings

Per serving: 365 calories, 10 g protein, 53 g carbohydrates, 14 g total fat, 1.5 g saturated fat, 3 g fiber, 599 mg sodium

Curried Pineapple Fried Rice

Prep Time: 15 minutes ★ **Total Time:** 30 minutes

Fried rice is always best made with cold leftover rice; with warm rice, it just gets mushy.

2 tablespoons light olive oil

1 onion, chopped

½ cup cashews, chopped

½ cup frozen peas

1 red bell pepper, chopped

1 clove garlic, minced

1 tablespoon minced fresh ginger

1 tablespoon curry powder

¾ teaspoon salt

2 cups leftover cooked brown rice or brown basmati rice

1 can (8 ounces) pineapple chunks in juice, drained

8 ounces firm tofu, drained and chopped

¼ cup finely chopped cilantro

1. Heat the oil in a large skillet over medium heat. Cook the onion for 5 minutes, or until tender. Stir in the cashews, peas, pepper, garlic, ginger, curry powder, and salt. Cook, stirring occasionally, for 2 minutes.

2. Stir in the rice. Cook for 5 minutes, stirring occasionally, until lightly browned. Stir in the pineapple and tofu and cook for 3 minutes, or until heated through.

3. Stir in the cilantro.

Makes 4 servings

Per serving: 373 calories, 12 g protein, 42 g carbohydrates, 18 g total fat, 3 g saturated fat, 6 g fiber, 449 mg sodium

Cheese Polenta with Mushrooms

Prep Time: 15 minutes ★ **Total Time:** 1 hour 5 minutes

You can make and bake the polenta ahead of time and refrigerate until ready to use. When it's time to serve it, cut the cold polenta into wedges, brush with a little olive oil, and broil or grill for 3 to 5 minutes, or until crusty and heated through.

Polenta

- 3 **cups water, divided**
- 1 **cup fine cornmeal**
- ¼ **cup extra-virgin olive oil**
- 1 **cup shredded reduced-fat Cheddar cheese**
- ⅓ **cup grated Parmesan cheese**
- ½ **teaspoon salt**

Topping

- 2 **tablespoons extra-virgin olive oil**
- 2 **large cloves garlic, minced**
- 8 **ounces white or baby bella mushrooms, trimmed and thinly sliced**
- 4 **ounces shiitake mushrooms, trimmed and thinly sliced**
- 1 **tablespoon chopped fresh rosemary or 1 teaspoon dried**
- ¼ **teaspoon salt**
- 2 **large tomatoes, cored, seeded, and chopped**

1. *To make the polenta:* Preheat the oven to 350°F. Lightly coat a 9" pie plate with cooking spray. Heat 2 cups of the water to a boil.

2. In a medium saucepan, combine the cornmeal and the remaining 1 cup water. Slowly pour in the boiling water, stirring constantly. Bring to a boil over medium heat. Cook, stirring, for 5 minutes, or until the mixture is bubbly and thick. Remove from the heat and stir in the oil, Cheddar, Parmesan, and salt. Spread into the pie plate.

3. Bake for 35 minutes, or until the top is crusty. Cut into 6 wedges.

4. *To make the topping:* Meanwhile, heat the oil in a large skillet over medium heat. Cook the garlic for 30 seconds. Add the white or baby bella mushrooms, shiitake mushrooms, rosemary, and salt. Cook, stirring occasionally, for 8 minutes, or until any liquid that collects in the skillet evaporates.

5. Stir in the tomatoes. Cook, stirring often, for 8 to 10 minutes, or until the tomatoes wilt and the mixture is heated through.

6. Place 1 wedge of the polenta on 6 plates. Divide the mushroom mixture over the polenta.

Makes 6 servings

Per serving: 293 calories, 10 g protein, 21 g carbohydrates, 19 g total fat, 5 g saturated fat, 4 g fiber, 495 mg sodium

Stuffed Chard Leaves

Prep Time: 45 minutes ★ **Total Time:** 2 hours

This is similar to a classic recipe for stuffed grape leaves but uses fresh greens instead. If you like, you can use an 8-ounce jar of grape leaves, rinsed and drained, in place of the chard and proceed with the recipe as directed, eliminating the boiling water rinse. Stuffed leaves can be used as a vegetarian main dish, an appetizer served with chunks of feta cheese on a party platter, or a side dish to accompany roast meat, cheese, or other vegetable dishes. The liquid remaining in the pan after the leaves are cooked is delicious drizzled over feta cheese, chickpeas and other legumes, or steamed vegetables such as green beans or asparagus.

½ cup extra-virgin olive oil, divided

1 onion, finely chopped

1 small fennel bulb, halved, cored, and chopped

2 cloves garlic, minced

1 teaspoon grated lemon peel

¾ cup brown rice

⅓ cup almonds, chopped

2 cups low-fat, reduced-sodium chicken or vegetable broth, divided

2 tablespoons finely chopped dill or 2 teaspoons dried

¼ cup finely chopped parsley

½ teaspoon salt

4 cups water

24 leaves chard, trimmed

½ cup lemon juice (from 3 lemons)

1. Heat ¼ cup of the oil in a large skillet over medium heat. Cook the onion, fennel, garlic, and lemon peel, stirring occasionally, for 10 minutes. Stir in the rice and almonds. Cook for 2 minutes, stirring often.

2. Add 1 cup of the broth. Reduce the heat to low, cover, and simmer for 25 minutes, or until all of the liquid is absorbed. Transfer to a medium bowl. Stir in the dill, parsley, and salt. Set aside to cool.

3. Meanwhile, bring the water to a boil. Place the chard in a colander in the sink. Pour the boiling water over the leaves so they wilt. When cool enough to handle, flatten the leaves and layer them on a plate or work surface.

4. Lay a leaf, dark side down, on the work surface. Spoon about 2 tablespoons of the rice mixture near the stem end. Fold the stem end up and over to cover the filling. Fold both sides of the leaf toward the middle, then continue to roll up the leaf, forming a snug bundle. Place the stuffed leaf, seam side down, in a deep 10" skillet. Repeat with the remaining leaves and filling, placing the bundles close against each other in the skillet.

5. Pour the remaining 1 cup broth and ¼ cup oil and the lemon juice over the leaves. Cover and simmer over low heat for 45 minutes, or until the bundles are tender and the rice is fully cooked.

6. Serve the stuffed leaves warm or at room temperature, drizzled with the liquid remaining in the pan.

Makes 6 servings

Per serving: 86 calories, 2 g protein, 8 g carbohydrates, 6 g total fat, 1 g saturated fat, 2 g fiber, 194 mg sodium

Tomato and Olive Roasted Fish

Prep Time: 10 minutes ★ **Total Time:** 30 minutes

Serve with a salad made with cold steamed asparagus and arugula, fresh basil, mushrooms, and olive oil vinaigrette.

1 pound blackfish, halibut, or other firm whitefish fillets

1 tablespoon olive oil, divided

½ teaspoon salt

¼ teaspoon ground black pepper

1½ cups cherry or grape tomatoes, halved

⅓ cup pitted imported olives, such as kalamata, finely chopped

¼ cup finely chopped flat-leaf parsley

1 large clove garlic, minced

2 teaspoons balsamic or red wine vinegar or lemon juice

1. Preheat the oven to 425°F. Lightly coat a rimmed baking sheet or shallow baking pan with cooking spray.

2. Rub the fish with 2 teaspoons of the oil. Place in a single layer in the pan. Sprinkle evenly with the salt and pepper.

3. Bake for 8 minutes.

4. Meanwhile, in a small bowl, combine the tomatoes, olives, parsley, garlic, vinegar or lemon juice, and the remaining 1 teaspoon oil. When the fish has baked for 8 minutes, carefully remove the pan from the oven, leaving the oven on. Spoon the tomato mixture evenly over the fillets and return the pan to the oven.

5. Bake for 5 to 10 minutes, or until the fish flakes easily. Serve at once.

Makes 4 servings

Per serving: 153 calories, 18 g protein, 4 g carbohydrates, 7 g total fat, 1 g saturated fat, 1 g fiber, 373 mg sodium

Oven-Fried Tilapia

Prep Time: 10 minutes ★ **Total Time:** 25 minutes

Serve with coleslaw or a chopped tomato and white bean salad, sprinkled with oregano and drizzled with olive oil vinaigrette.

½ **cup fresh whole wheat bread crumbs (see note)**

¼ **cup fine cornmeal**

½ **teaspoon salt**

¼ **teaspoon ground black pepper**

½ **cup low-fat plain yogurt**

2 **tablespoons lemon juice**

1 **pound tilapia fillets, cut in 4 equal pieces**

1. Preheat the oven to 425°F. Lightly coat a baking sheet with cooking spray.

2. On a plate, combine the bread crumbs, cornmeal, salt, and pepper.

3. In a medium bowl, combine the yogurt and lemon juice.

4. Dip the tilapia in the yogurt mixture, then coat both sides with the crumb mixture and place on the prepared baking sheet.

5. Bake for 10 to 15 minutes, or until the fish flakes easily.

NOTE: To make ½ cup of fresh crumbs, process 1 slice whole wheat bread in a food processor until fine crumbs form.

Makes 4 servings

Per serving: 159 calories, 24 g protein, 12 g carbohydrates, 2 g total fat, 1 g saturated fat, 2 g fiber, 383 mg sodium

Salmon Cakes with Cucumber Dressing

Prep Time: 25 minutes ★ **Total Time:** 45 minutes

Serve these salmon cakes on a bed of baby arugula or mixed baby greens dressed with olive oil vinaigrette, accompanied by barley or brown rice and sautéed mushrooms.

Dressing

- 2 cucumbers, peeled, halved lengthwise, seeded, and thinly sliced
- ¼ cup low-fat plain yogurt
- ¼ teaspoon salt

Salmon Cakes

- 1¼ pounds salmon fillet, skinned and finely chopped
- 1 cup whole wheat bread crumbs (see note)
- 2 ribs celery, finely chopped
- 2 scallions, finely chopped
- 1 red bell pepper, finely chopped
- 1 egg
- 2 tablespoons Dijon mustard
- ½ teaspoon salt
- 2 tablespoons extra-virgin olive oil, divided

1. *To make the dressing:* In a medium bowl, combine the cucumbers and yogurt. Refrigerate until ready to serve. Just before serving, stir in the salt.

2. *To make the salmon cakes:* In a large bowl, combine the salmon, bread crumbs, celery, scallions, bell pepper, egg, mustard, and salt. Stir until well combined. Shape into 8 patties.

3. Heat 1 tablespoon of the oil in a large skillet over medium-high heat. Cook 4 salmon cakes for 6 minutes, turning once, or until browned and the salmon is opaque in the center. Transfer to a platter and cover to keep warm. Repeat with the remaining oil and salmon cakes. Serve with the cucumber dressing.

NOTE: To make ½ cup of fresh crumbs, process 1 slice whole wheat bread in a food processor until fine crumbs form.

Makes 8 servings

Per serving: 184 calories, 17 g protein, 8 g carbohydrates, 9 g total fat, 1 g saturated fat, 2 g fiber, 400 mg sodium

Scallop and Grape Tomato Sauté

Prep Time: 5 minutes ★ **Total Time:** 10 minutes

This is a great dinner for a busy weeknight, because it can be prepared from start to finish in less than 10 minutes! You can use baby spinach or watercress instead of the arugula. Serve with whole wheat orzo or other whole wheat pasta, quick-cooking brown rice, or crusty whole wheat Italian bread.

2 tablespoons extra-virgin olive oil

1 pound sea scallops

2 cups grape tomatoes, halved

2 cloves garlic, minced

½ teaspoon dried oregano

½ teaspoon salt

⅛ teaspoon red-pepper flakes (optional)

4 cups baby arugula

1. Heat the oil in a large nonstick skillet over medium-high heat. Add the scallops and cook for 2 minutes, turning once, or until browned.

2. Add the tomatoes, garlic, oregano, salt, and pepper flakes (if using). Cook, stirring occasionally, for 1 minute, or until the tomatoes start to soften.

3. Add the arugula and cook, stirring, for 1 minute, or until the arugula wilts and the scallops are opaque.

Makes 4 servings

Per serving: 184 calories, 20 g protein, 7 g carbohydrates, 8 g total fat, 1 g saturated fat, 1 g fiber, 483 mg sodium

Shrimp with Garlic, Basil, and Fennel

Prep Time: 15 minutes ★ **Total Time:** 30 minutes

Serve with whole grain angel hair pasta and sautéed zucchini with grated Parmesan cheese.

2 tablespoons extra-virgin olive oil

1 small onion, halved and thinly sliced

1 large clove garlic, minced

1 fennel bulb, trimmed, cored, and thinly sliced

¾ pound peeled, deveined large shrimp

½ cup fresh basil leaves

2 tablespoons balsamic vinegar

½ teaspoon salt

1. Heat the oil in a large skillet over medium heat. Cook the onion for 5 minutes, or until lightly browned. Add the garlic and cook for 1 minute. Stir in the fennel and cook for 3 minutes. Add the shrimp and cook, stirring often, for 2 minutes, or until opaque.

2. Meanwhile, stack the basil leaves on top of each other and roll up tightly from 1 long side. Cut crosswise into thin slices.

3. Stir in the vinegar, basil, and salt.

Makes 4 servings

Per serving: 173 calories, 16 g protein, 8 g carbohydrates, 8 g total fat, 1 g saturated fat, 2 g fiber, 429 mg sodium

Grilled Fish and Vegetable Kebabs

Prep Time: 15 minutes ★ **Total Time:** 25 minutes + marinating time

Try with wild rice and coleslaw or a mixed green salad.

3 tablespoons extra-virgin olive oil

3 tablespoons red wine vinegar

2 large cloves garlic, minced

2 teaspoons dried tarragon

1 teaspoon Dijon mustard

8 button or baby bella mushrooms

1 green bell pepper, cut into 8 pieces

1 red, orange, or yellow bell pepper, cut into 8 pieces

1 red onion, cut into 8 wedges

1¼ pounds halibut, tuna, scrod, bluefish, or salmon, cut into 16 chunks (1"–1¼" thick)

1. In a large bowl, whisk together the oil, vinegar, garlic, tarragon, and mustard.

2. Add the mushrooms and peppers and toss well. Carefully stir in the onion wedges so they don't fall apart. Marinate for at least 30 minutes or up to 2 hours. Add the fish to the marinade 15 minutes before you are ready to cook.

3. Preheat the broiler or grill.

4. On each of eight (12") skewers, thread 1 mushroom, 1 chunk of fish, 1 piece of green pepper, 1 onion wedge, another chunk of fish, and 1 piece of red, orange, or yellow pepper. Discard the remaining marinade.

5. Broil or grill for 8 minutes, turning once, or until the vegetables are singed and the fish flakes easily.

Makes 4 servings

Per serving: 287 calories, 31 g protein, 7 g carbohydrates, 14 g total fat, 2 g saturated fat, 2 g fiber, 112 mg sodium

Veggie-Stuffed Meat Loaf

Prep Time: 20 minutes ★ **Total Time:** 1 hour

Although Mediterranean cooking emphasizes fresh vegetables for their great flavor and abundance of valuable nutrients, frozen spinach and bottled peppers will do here in a pinch. If you don't have leftover rice or bulgur to use as a binder, add 1 cup instant or quick-cooking oats instead. Serve with a tomato-olive salad and roasted new potatoes.

1 tablespoon olive oil

1 onion, finely chopped

4 cups fresh spinach leaves (baby spinach works well)

1 roasted red pepper, chopped

2 cloves garlic, minced

12 ounces extra-lean ground beef, turkey, or a combination of lean ground meats

1 cup cooked brown rice or bulgur

½ teaspoon dried thyme

¼ teaspoon salt

1 cup shredded reduced-fat Cheddar cheese

¼ cup no-salt-added ketchup

1 tablespoon balsamic vinegar

1. Preheat the oven to 400°F.

2. Heat the oil in a large skillet over medium heat. Cook the onion for 5 minutes, or until tender. Stir in the spinach, pepper, and garlic. Cook for 1 minute, or until the spinach wilts.

3. In a large bowl, combine the meat, rice or bulgur, thyme, and the salt until well mixed.

4. On a piece of foil, pat the meat mixture out into a ½"-thick rectangle. Sprinkle with the cheese to within ½" of the edges of the meat. Spread the vegetable mixture over the cheese.

5. Using the foil, carefully roll up the meat loaf from 1 long side, jelly-roll style, ending with the seam side against the foil. Transfer to a rimmed baking sheet or medium roasting pan.

6. In a small bowl, combine the ketchup and vinegar. Brush evenly over the meat loaf.

7. Bake for 30 to 35 minutes, or until a thermometer inserted in the center registers 160°F and the meat is no longer pink. Let stand for 10 minutes before cutting into 8 slices.

Makes 4 servings

Per serving: 319 calories, 27 g protein, 20 g carbohydrates, 13 g total fat, 5.5 g saturated fat, 3 g fiber, 562 mg sodium

Orange Beef Stir-Fry

Prep Time: 10 minutes ★ **Total Time:** 20 minutes + marinating time

Serve over brown rice, with a cucumber and watercress salad on the side.

2 teaspoons cornstarch

¼ cup orange juice

2 tablespoons light soy sauce

1 tablespoon honey

1 tablespoon grated orange peel

12 ounces beef sirloin, top round, or flank steak, thinly sliced

1 tablespoon light olive oil

3 cloves garlic, minced

1 tablespoon minced fresh ginger

2 cups snow peas

1. In a medium bowl, stir together the cornstarch, orange juice, soy sauce, honey, and orange peel until well blended. Add the beef and toss to coat with the marinade. Set aside for 15 minutes.

2. Heat the oil in a large skillet or wok over medium-high heat. Cook the garlic and ginger, stirring constantly, for 1 minute. Add the reserved beef with the marinade. Cook, stirring often, for 3 to 5 minutes, or until all of the meat is browned.

3. Add the snow peas and cook, stirring, for 1 minute.

Makes 4 servings

Per serving: 202 calories, 17 g protein, 11 g carbohydrates, 10 g total fat, 3 g saturated fat, 1 g fiber, 350 mg sodium

Lamb Stew with Chickpeas and Bulgur

Prep Time: 15 minutes ★ **Total Time:** 2 hours 5 minutes

If you're not a lamb fan, you can make this dish with beef stew meat. Freeze any leftovers for another meal. Serve with a crisp salad topped with grilled zucchini.

¼ cup olive oil

1 pound lamb for stew or lean lamb shoulder, cut into 1" cubes

1 large onion, chopped

4 cloves garlic, minced

2 teaspoons ground cumin

1 can (14.5 ounces) low-fat, reduced-sodium beef or chicken broth

1 can (14.5 ounces) diced tomatoes

2 cups water

1 can (15 ounces) no-salt-added chickpeas, drained

½ cup bulgur

4 cups fresh baby spinach

1. Heat the oil in a large saucepan over medium-high heat. Cook the lamb for 10 minutes, stirring, or until browned on all sides. Use a slotted spoon to transfer the lamb to a bowl and set aside.

2. Add the onion, garlic, and cumin to the pan. Reduce the heat to medium and cook for 5 minutes, stirring occasionally, or until the onion is lightly browned.

3. Stir in the lamb, broth, and tomatoes. Cover, reduce the heat to medium-low, and simmer for 1 hour.

4. Stir in the water, chickpeas, and bulgur. Bring to a boil over medium-high heat. Reduce the heat to medium-low, cover, and simmer for 30 minutes, or until the bulgur is tender and fluffy.

5. Stir in the spinach. Simmer for 5 minutes.

Makes 8 servings

Per serving: 285 calories, 16 g protein, 22 g carbohydrates, 15 g total fat, 4 g saturated fat, 5 g fiber, 290 mg sodium

Roasted Pork Tenderloin and Peppers with Arugula Pesto

Prep Time: 10 minutes ★ **Total Time:** 40 minutes

Serve this dish with whole wheat couscous or brown rice. The unusual but delicious pesto is also great tossed with whole wheat pasta.

Pork and Peppers

¾ pound pork tenderloin

3 bell peppers, quartered

1 tablespoon extra-virgin olive oil

½ teaspoon salt

¼ teaspoon ground black pepper

Pesto

2 cups baby arugula

¼ cup extra-virgin olive oil

¼ cup water

¼ cup blanched almonds

1 clove garlic

¼ teaspoon salt

1. *To make the pork and peppers:* Preheat the oven to 475°F. Coat a large rimmed baking sheet with cooking spray. Place the pork and bell peppers on the pan, brush with the oil, and sprinkle with the salt and black pepper.

2. Roast for 25 to 30 minutes, or until a thermometer inserted in the center of the pork reaches 145°F and the juices run clear. Let the pork stand for 5 minutes before slicing.

3. *To make the pesto:* Meanwhile, in a blender or food processor, combine the arugula, oil, water, almonds, garlic, and salt. Process until smooth. Serve with the sliced pork and peppers.

Makes 4 servings

Per serving: 325 calories, 21 g protein, 7 g carbohydrates, 24 g total fat, 3.5 g saturated fat, 3 g fiber, 490 mg sodium

Rescue Vinaigrette

Prep Time: 5 minutes ★ **Total Time:** 5 minutes

You can use this delicious and easy-to-make dressing on your salad every day on the Diabetes Rescue Diet. Pick a variation and enjoy a tablespoon or two to make sure you're getting enough antioxidant-rich EVOO in your diet.

⅓ cup extra-virgin olive oil

2 tablespoons red or white wine vinegar

⅛ teaspoon salt

⅛ teaspoon ground black pepper

In a small bowl, whisk together the oil, vinegar, salt, and pepper. Cover and refrigerate until ready to serve.

VARIATIONS:

Garlic: Add 1 clove crushed or minced garlic.

Herb: Add 1 tablespoon finely chopped fresh or ½ teaspoon dried basil, cilantro, dill, oregano, parsley, tarragon, or thyme.

Mustard: Add ¼ teaspoon Dijon mustard.

Onion: Add 1 tablespoon finely chopped scallion or red onion.

Lemon: Substitute 3 tablespoons lemon juice for the 2 tablespoons vinegar.

Curry: Prepare lemon vinaigrette and add ¼ teaspoon curry powder.

Creamy: Add 1 tablespoon low-fat plain yogurt.

Makes 4 servings (2 tablespoons each)

Per serving: 168 calories, 0 g protein, 0 g carbohydrates, 19 g total fat, 2.5 g saturated fat, 0 g fiber, 73 mg sodium

Butter Beans in Fresh Tomato Sauce

Prep Time: 10 minutes ★ **Total Time:** 30 minutes

You can substitute cannellini or navy beans for the butter beans, if you like.

2 tablespoons extra-virgin olive oil

1 onion, finely chopped

2 tablespoons minced garlic

2 large tomatoes, cored, seeded, and chopped

1 tablespoon finely chopped fresh sage or 1 teaspoon dried

¼ teaspoon salt

1 can (14–19 ounces) butter beans, rinsed and drained

1. Heat the oil in a large skillet over medium heat. Cook the onion for 5 minutes, or until lightly browned. Add the garlic and cook for 1 minute.

2. Stir in the tomatoes, sage, and salt. Cook, stirring occasionally, for 5 minutes, or until the tomatoes are softened. Stir in the beans and cook for 5 minutes, or until heated through.

Makes 4 servings

Per serving: 113 calories, 1 g protein, 8 g carbohydrates, 8 g total fat, 1 g saturated fat, 2 g fiber, 151 mg sodium

Refried Beans

Prep Time: 10 minutes ★ **Total Time:** 25 minutes

Mashed beans go with any Tex-Mex meal or as a side dish with roasted meats. Making them yourself allows you to control the type of fat and amount of salt used. These lightly seasoned beans are also more flavorful than most commercial varieties.

2 tablespoons extra-virgin olive oil

1 clove garlic, minced

½ teaspoon chili powder

¼ teaspoon ground cumin

2 cans (14–19 ounces each) no-salt-added pinto beans, undrained

½ teaspoon salt

¼ cup finely chopped cilantro (optional)

1. Heat the oil in a large skillet over medium heat. Add the garlic, chili powder, and cumin and cook, stirring, for 1 minute. Stir in the beans (with their liquid) and salt.

2. Use a potato masher or the back of a large spoon to mash the beans until they are the consistency of mashed potatoes. Cook for 10 minutes, or until heated through.

3. Remove from the heat and stir in the cilantro (if using).

Makes 8 servings

Per serving: 109 calories, 5 g protein, 14 g carbohydrates, 4 g total fat, 0.5 g saturated fat, 5 g fiber, 157 mg sodium

Wilted Garlicky Greens

Prep Time: 15 minutes ★ **Total Time:** 30 minutes

Leafy green vegetables are available year-round and are especially abundant in summertime. Use plenty of garlic and a combination of at least 2 or 3 greens for the best flavor.

3 tablespoons extra-virgin olive oil

1 large onion, finely chopped

4 cloves garlic, minced

1 tablespoon finely chopped fresh ginger

6 cups coarsely chopped or torn mixed greens, such as Swiss chard, arugula, or spinach or beet, dandelion, or mustard greens

½ teaspoon salt

¼ teaspoon ground black pepper

1. Heat the oil in a large saucepan over medium heat. Cook the onion for 5 minutes, or until lightly browned. Add the garlic and ginger and cook for 30 seconds.

2. Stir in the greens, salt, and pepper. Cover the pan and cook for 5 minutes, or until the greens wilt.

Makes 4 servings

Per serving: 127 calories, 2 g protein, 7 g carbohydrates, 11 g total fat, 1.5 g saturated fat, 2 g fiber, 405 mg sodium

Wild Rice and Barley Pilaf

Prep Time: 10 minutes ★ **Total Time:** 1 hour 5 minutes

Hearty grains go well with meat or with egg and cheese dishes such as quiche.

1 tablespoon extra-virgin olive oil, divided

1 large onion, finely chopped

½ cup wild rice or unseasoned wild and brown rice mixture

⅓ cup regular barley

1 can (14.5 ounces) low-fat, reduced-sodium chicken or vegetable broth

1 cup water

8 ounces mushrooms, trimmed and thinly sliced

½ cup walnuts

1 teaspoon dried thyme, crumbled

½ teaspoon salt

1. Heat 2 teaspoons of the oil in a large saucepan over medium heat. Cook the onion for 5 minutes, or until lightly browned. Add the rice and barley. Cook, stirring often, for 2 minutes.

2. Stir in the broth and water. Heat to a boil over medium-high heat. Reduce the heat to low, cover, and simmer for 45 minutes, or until the grains are tender and the liquid is absorbed.

3. Meanwhile, heat the remaining 1 teaspoon oil in a medium nonstick skillet over medium heat. Cook the mushrooms for 10 minutes, or until tender and any liquid in the pan has evaporated. Stir in the walnuts, thyme, and salt. Cook, stirring occasionally, for 2 minutes. Stir into the rice mixture.

Makes 8 servings

Per serving: 142 calories, 5 g protein, 17 g carbohydrates, 7 g total fat, 1 g saturated fat, 3 g fiber, 263 mg sodium

Roasted Peppers with Capers and Anchovies

Prep Time: 15 minutes ★ **Total Time:** 15 minutes

Delicious as a side dish with meat, poultry, or fish or a rice or pasta entrée, this mixture is also good finely chopped and used as a topping for very thinly sliced and toasted whole grain Italian bread or baguette. You can also add it to a green salad.

1 clove garlic

2 anchovies

1 tablespoon extra-virgin olive oil

2 teaspoons drained capers

¼ teaspoon salt

⅛ teaspoon ground black pepper

3 large roasted red peppers, cut into thick lengthwise slices

¼ cup thinly sliced fresh basil or 1 teaspoon dried, crumbled

1. Rub the inside of a medium bowl with the garlic. Add the anchovies and oil and mash together until smooth. Stir in the capers, salt, and black pepper.

2. Add the roasted peppers and basil and toss to coat well.

Makes 4 servings

Per serving: 60 calories, 3 g protein, 2 g carbohydrates, 4 g total fat, 1 g saturated fat, 0 g fiber, 317 mg sodium

Broiled Tomatoes with Curry

Prep Time: 10 minutes ★ **Total Time:** 20 minutes

Serve alongside meat, poultry, or seafood or any type of bean dish.

4 **large plum tomatoes, halved lengthwise**

¼ **teaspoon salt**

⅛ **teaspoon ground black pepper**

2 **teaspoons extra-virgin olive oil**

¼ **cup mayonnaise**

¼ **cup 0% plain Greek yogurt**

½ **teaspoon curry powder**

1. Preheat the broiler. Set an oven rack so it is 6" from the heat source. Coat a broiler pan with cooking spray.

2. Remove the seeds from the tomato halves. Arrange the halves, cut side up, on the pan. Sprinkle evenly with the salt and pepper. Drizzle each half with ¼ teaspoon of the oil.

3. Broil for 5 minutes.

4. Meanwhile, in a small bowl, combine the mayonnaise, yogurt, and curry powder. Spread evenly over the tomatoes.

5. Broil for 1 to 2 minutes, or until the mayonnaise is lightly browned.

Makes 4 servings

Per serving: 141 calories, 2 g protein, 3 g carbohydrates, 13 g total fat, 2 g saturated fat, 1 g fiber, 244 mg sodium

Pineapple Roasted Sweet Potatoes

Prep Time: 10 minutes ★ **Total Time:** 1 hour

This is an especially good dish for the holidays. Serve with roast meat or poultry and sautéed broccoli rabe or other leafy greens.

2 large sweet potatoes, peeled and cut into 1½" chunks

3 tablespoons extra-virgin olive oil

4 cloves garlic, thinly sliced

1 tablespoon finely chopped fresh ginger

½ teaspoon ground cumin

½ teaspoon salt

2 cups fresh 1" pineapple cubes

½ cup chopped walnuts

1 tablespoon honey

1. Preheat the oven to 400°F.

2. In a 13" × 9" baking dish, combine the potatoes, oil, garlic, ginger, cumin, and salt. Toss to coat well.

3. Bake for 20 minutes, stirring occasionally.

4. Meanwhile, in a medium bowl, combine the pineapple, walnuts, and honey. Stir into the potatoes. Bake for 30 minutes, or until the mixture is browned and the potatoes are tender.

Makes 6 servings

Per serving: 259 calories, 4 g protein, 33 g carbohydrates, 14 g total fat, 1.5 g saturated fat, 5 g fiber, 253 mg sodium

Orange Fennel Slaw

Prep Time: 20 minutes ★ **Total Time:** 20 minutes

If you can't find fresh fennel, substitute an equal amount of celery or thinly sliced red bell pepper. The licorice-like flavor of raw fennel goes well with seafood and tomato dishes.

2 tablespoons extra-virgin olive oil

2 tablespoons white wine vinegar

2 tablespoons low-fat plain yogurt

1 tablespoon mayonnaise

2 teaspoons Dijon mustard

1 teaspoon fennel seeds, crushed (optional)

¾ teaspoon salt

4 cups shredded green cabbage

2 cups shredded red cabbage

1 fennel bulb, halved, and thinly sliced

1 orange, cut into sections or 1 can (15 ounces) no-sugar-added mandarin oranges

½ cup sliced fresh basil leaves (see note)

1. In a large bowl, whisk together the oil, vinegar, yogurt, mayonnaise, mustard, fennel seeds (if using), and salt.

2. Add the green cabbage, red cabbage, fennel, orange sections, and basil. Toss well.

NOTE: To slice basil, stack several leaves on top of each other. Roll up tightly from 1 long side. Cut crosswise into thin slices.

Makes 8 servings

Per serving: 77 calories, 1 g protein, 8 g carbohydrates, 5 g total fat, 1 g saturated fat, 3 g fiber, 286 mg sodium

Roasted Vegetables

Prep Time: 20 minutes ★ **Total Time:** 50 minutes

You can also roast broccoli florets, bell pepper and onion chunks, zucchini, and even green beans. You may have to adjust cooking times for different vegetables, but the basic recipe and method are the same.

½ **head cauliflower, cut into florets**

1 **pint Brussels sprouts, halved**

2 **cups baby carrots, halved lengthwise**

4 **large cloves garlic, halved and sliced**

2 **tablespoons extra-virgin olive oil**

2 **tablespoons lemon juice**

2 **tablespoons fresh chopped sage or 1 tablespoon dried**

½ **teaspoon salt**

¼ **teaspoon ground black pepper**

1. Preheat the oven to 425°F.

2. In a 13" × 9" baking dish, combine the cauliflower, Brussels sprouts, carrots, and garlic. Drizzle with the oil and lemon juice. Sprinkle with the sage, salt, and pepper. Gently toss to combine and coat all the vegetables with the oil and seasonings.

3. Roast for 15 minutes. Stir the vegetables. Roast for 10 to 15 minutes, or until the vegetables are tender-crisp and browned around the edges. Serve at once.

Makes 8 servings

Per serving: 67 calories, 2 g protein, 8 g carbohydrates, 4 g total fat, 0.5 g saturated fat, 2 g fiber, 177 mg sodium

Quick Marinated Vegetables

Prep Time: 30 minutes ★ **Total Time:** 45 minutes

Enjoy these crisp, tasty vegetables as you would a side dish or salad. Serve them just after marinating, or make them ahead of time for a later meal.

¾ cup distilled white vinegar

¼ cup wine vinegar, such as sherry, balsamic, white, or red

4 cloves garlic

1 teaspoon sugar or equivalent sugar substitute

½ teaspoon salt

½ teaspoon black peppercorns

½ head cauliflower or broccoli, cut into florets

1 zucchini, halved lengthwise and cut into ½"-thick slices

1 large red or green bell pepper, cut into bite-size chunks

1 small red onion, cut into 8 wedges

2 sprigs fresh thyme or 1 teaspoon dried

½ cup extra-virgin olive oil

1. In a medium saucepan, heat the white vinegar, wine vinegar, garlic, sugar, salt, and peppercorns over medium heat, just until the mixture comes to a boil.

2. In a large bowl, combine the cauliflower or broccoli, zucchini, bell pepper, onion, and thyme. Pour the hot vinegar mixture over the vegetables. Add the oil and toss to coat.

3. Let stand for 15 minutes, stirring often, before serving. Cover and refrigerate any remaining vegetables in the marinade for up to 5 days, stirring occasionally.

Makes 12 servings

Per serving: 103 calories, 1 g protein, 4 g carbohydrates, 9 g total fat, 1 g saturated fat, 1 g fiber, 107 mg sodium

Pita Scoops

Prep Time: 20 minutes ★ **Total Time:** 35 minutes

You can easily double this recipe if you're having a party. Make the pita chips slightly ahead of time and the topping just before serving.

4 **small whole wheat pitas, cut into quarters**

1 **egg white**

2 **tablespoons extra-virgin olive oil**

2 **tablespoons grated Parmesan cheese**

2 **cloves garlic, minced**

½ **teaspoon dried oregano, crumbled**

½ **cup finely chopped cucumber**

¼ **cup finely chopped tomato**

6 **kalamata olives, finely chopped**

2 **tablespoons feta cheese**

2 **tablespoons 2% plain Greek yogurt**

1. Preheat the oven to 300°F. Lightly coat a large baking sheet with cooking spray.

2. Pull each pita wedge apart to form a total of 32 triangles. Place on the baking sheet.

3. In a small bowl, whisk together the egg white, oil, Parmesan, garlic, and oregano. Brush evenly on the inside of the pita triangles.

4. Bake for 15 minutes, or until the seasoning is set and the edges of the triangles are lightly browned. Cool on a rack.

5. Meanwhile, in a small bowl, combine the cucumber, tomato, olives, feta cheese, and yogurt. Spoon about 1 tablespoon of cucumber mixture onto each pita chip, or use the chips to scoop the topping from the bowl.

Makes 8 servings

Per serving: 96 calories, 3 g protein, 9 g carbohydrates, 6 g total fat, 1 g saturated fat, 1 g fiber, 174 mg sodium

Hummus

Prep Time: 15 minutes ★ **Total Time:** 15 minutes

Although prepared hummus is widely available in supermarkets, the fresh taste of homemade makes it worth preparing yourself. If you're a real do-it-yourself cook, you can even prepare the chickpeas from scratch (see note). Serve with vegetable dippers and toasted wedges of whole grain pita. For variations, add 1 roasted pepper, 1 cup drained marinated artichokes, ½ cup kalamata olives, or ½ cup drained canned beets when processing the chickpea mixture, or substitute 1 cup cooked edamame (green soybeans) or other beans for 1 cup chickpeas.

3 **large cloves garlic**

1 **can (15–19 ounces) no-salt-added chickpeas**

¾ **cup tahini (sesame paste)**

½ **cup lemon juice (from 3 lemons)**

⅓ **cup water**

½ **teaspoon salt**

1 **tablespoon extra-virgin olive oil**

¼ **cup chopped parsley**

1. Process the garlic in a food processor or blender until finely chopped. Add the chickpeas, tahini, lemon juice, water, and salt. Process until very smooth, adding a little more water, if necessary.

2. Place in a serving bowl. Pour the oil over the top and sprinkle with the parsley. Serve at once, or cover and refrigerate for up to 8 hours before serving.

NOTE: To make hummus from dried chickpeas, soak 1¼ cups dried chickpeas overnight in enough water to cover. Drain and place in a medium saucepan with fresh water to cover by 1". Bring to a boil over medium-high heat. Reduce the heat to low, cover, and simmer for 1½ hours, or until the chickpeas crush easily with a fork. Drain, cool, and continue with the recipe as directed.

Makes 8 servings

Per serving: 218 calories, 9 g protein, 13 g carbohydrates, 16 g total fat, 2 g saturated fat, 3 g fiber, 155 mg sodium

Smoked Salmon Dip

Prep Time: 10 minutes ★ **Total Time:** 10 minutes

If you would rather have a spread than a dip, prepare the recipe by hand rather than in a food processor, and stir the yogurt in near the end so you can better control the consistency. Serve with cucumber and radish slices, bell pepper strips, or cherry tomatoes on picks.

8 ounces reduced-fat cream cheese

½ cup 0% plain Greek yogurt

1 tablespoon lemon juice

1 teaspoon prepared horseradish

1 teaspoon Dijon mustard

1 tablespoon chopped fresh dill or 1 teaspoon dried

4 ounces smoked salmon (or other smoked fish, such as trout or bluefish)

¼ cup finely chopped red onion (optional)

1 tablespoon chopped capers (optional)

1. In a food processor, combine the cream cheese, yogurt, lemon juice, horseradish, mustard, and dill. Process until smooth. Add the salmon and process just until incorporated.

2. Place in a small bowl. Garnish with the onion and capers (if using) and serve, or cover and refrigerate for up to 48 hours.

Makes 8 servings

Per serving: 96 calories, 12 g protein, 1 g carbohydrates, 5 g total fat, 3 g saturated fat, 0 g fiber, 305 mg sodium

Tuna Pâté

Prep Time: 10 minutes ★ **Total Time:** 10 minutes

Spread on toasted thin slices of whole grain baguette or Italian bread or on sliced cucumber or chunks of bell pepper.

2 large cloves garlic

1 can (14–19 ounces) no-salt-added white beans, such as cannellini or great Northern, rinsed and drained

2 cans (7 ounces) tuna packed in water, well drained

¼ cup fresh parsley

3 tablespoons lemon juice

1 tablespoon extra-virgin olive oil

1 tablespoon chopped rosemary

1 tablespoon drained capers

½ teaspoon salt

⅛ teaspoon ground black pepper

1. Process the garlic in a food processor until minced. Add the beans, tuna, parsley, lemon juice, oil, rosemary, capers, salt, and pepper. Process just until smooth.

2. Place in a serving bowl. Cover and refrigerate if not serving immediately.

Makes 8 servings

Per serving: 99 calories, 12 g protein, 5 g carbohydrates, 3 g total fat, 1 g saturated fat, 1 g fiber, 210 mg sodium

Goat Cheese and Spinach Quesadillas

Prep Time: 10 minutes ★ **Total Time:** 15 minutes

You can reheat these quesadillas on a plate in a microwave oven. In a pinch, you can use 5 ounces (½ box) thawed and drained frozen spinach or other greens instead of fresh. If you want to serve the quesadillas as a lunch or dinner, the recipe makes 2 servings.

2 tablespoons extra-virgin olive oil

2 cloves garlic, minced

4 cups fresh baby spinach, arugula, or torn Swiss chard leaves

½ cup chopped roasted red pepper

4 ounces goat cheese

2 large (10") multigrain wraps made with extra-virgin olive oil

1. Heat the oil in a large skillet over medium heat. Cook the garlic, stirring, for 30 seconds. Add the spinach, arugula, or Swiss chard and cook, stirring, for 1 to 2 minutes, or until wilted. Remove from the heat and stir in the pepper.

2. Spread half of the goat cheese over half of 1 wrap. Top with half of the spinach mixture. Fold the unfilled half over the mixture. Repeat to make another quesadilla.

3. Carefully wipe or rinse out the skillet and heat over medium-high heat. Cook each quesadilla for 2 minutes, turning once, or until the wrap is crisp and lightly browned. Transfer to a cutting board to cut in half.

Makes 4 servings

Per serving: 206 calories, 10 g protein, 13 g carbohydrates, 14 g total fat, 5 g saturated fat, 5 g fiber, 409 mg sodium

Garlic-Parmesan Kale Chips

Prep Time: 15 minutes ★ **Total Time:** 35 minutes

To save time, you can use bottled garlic-flavored olive oil instead of making your own. If you do make the oil yourself, you can double or quadruple the ingredients and refrigerate the extra for up to a week, for use in cooking and on salads.

1½ **tablespoons extra-virgin olive oil**

1 **clove garlic, sliced**

6 **cups torn kale leaves (stems removed and well dried)**

1 **tablespoon grated Parmesan cheese**

¼ **teaspoon kosher salt**

1. In a microwaveable custard cup, combine the oil and garlic. Microwave on high power for 20 seconds, or until sizzling. Remove and set aside for at least 10 minutes.

2. Preheat the oven to 300°F. Place the kale on a large rimmed baking sheet. Remove and discard the garlic from the oil. Drizzle the oil over the kale. Using your hands, toss the kale and gently rub the oil into the leaves until evenly coated. Spread out into a single layer.

3. Bake for 15 to 20 minutes, or until the leaves are crisp but still green.

4. Remove from the oven and sprinkle with the cheese and salt.

Makes 4 servings

Per serving: 104 calories, 4 g protein, 10 g carbohydrates, 6 g total fat, 1 g saturated fat, 2 g fiber, 182 mg sodium

Crispy Tuscan-Roasted Chickpeas

Prep Time: 18 minutes ★ **Total Time:** 1 hour 5 minutes

The classic Tuscan flavors of fennel and rosemary perk up these addictive high-fiber snacks. They're so good, you might want to double the recipe, which can easily be done on the same baking sheet. Be sure to store any leftovers in an airtight container so they keep crisp.

1 can (14–19 ounces) chickpeas, rinsed and drained

1 tablespoon extra-virgin olive oil

2 teaspoons dried rosemary, crumbled

2 teaspoons fennel seeds, crushed

¼ teaspoon kosher salt

¼ teaspoon ground black pepper

1. Line a rimmed baking sheet with paper towels. Spread the chickpeas on top and let dry for 15 minutes. Pat dry with additional paper towels and discard any loose skins.

2. Meanwhile, preheat the oven to 400°F. In a large bowl, stir together the oil, rosemary, fennel seeds, salt, and pepper.

3. Add the chickpeas to the bowl and toss to coat. Remove and discard the paper towel from the baking sheet. Spread the chickpeas on the sheet and roast, tossing twice, for 35 to 45 minutes, or until dried, golden, and crisp. Let cool completely on the baking sheet on a wire rack, then serve or store in an airtight container.

Makes 4 servings

Per serving: 115 calories, 3 g protein, 15 g carbohydrates, 5 g total fat, 0.5 g saturated fat, 4 g fiber, 314 mg sodium

Peach-Almond Frostie

Prep Time: 10 minutes ★ **Total Time:** 10 minutes

A frostie is an icy smoothie made with crushed ice or frozen fruit. If it's not peach season, use 2 cups of frozen peaches and skip the ice cubes. If your peaches are very ripe, you probably won't need the honey.

2 ripe peaches, sliced

1½ cups unsweetened vanilla-almond beverage

¼ cup sliced natural almonds

2 tablespoons honey (optional)

4 ice cubes, cracked or crushed (see note)

1. In a blender, combine the peaches, almond beverage, almonds, honey (if using), and ice. Blend until smooth and icy.

2. Pour into 2 tall glasses.

NOTE: If you don't have an ice crusher, crack the ice cubes by placing them in a plastic bag and banging gently with a mallet or the bottom of a skillet.

Makes 2 servings

Per serving: 156 calories, 4 g protein, 19 g carbohydrates, 8 g total fat, 0.5 g saturated fat, 4 g fiber, 135 mg sodium

Herbed Cream Cheese

Prep Time: 10 minutes ★ **Total Time:** 10 minutes

You can spread this herb-infused cream cheese in mushroom caps or on pepper wedges, cucumber rounds, celery sticks, or whole grain crackers or toast. Like most seasoned cheese mixtures, this tastes even better the next day, when the flavors have had time to marry.

8 ounces reduced-fat cream cheese, at room temperature

2 tablespoons mayonnaise

2 tablespoons grated Parmesan cheese

1 clove garlic, minced

1 tablespoon finely chopped fresh dill or 1 teaspoon dried

2 teaspoons finely chopped fresh basil or ½ teaspoon dried

½ teaspoon finely chopped fresh thyme or ⅛ teaspoon dried

⅛ teaspoon ground black pepper

In a small bowl, combine the cream cheese, mayonnaise, Parmesan, garlic, dill, basil, thyme, and pepper.

Makes 16 servings (1 tablespoon each)

Per serving: 42 calories, 2 g protein, 1 g carbohydrates, 4 g total fat, 1.5 g saturated fat, 0 g fiber, 87 mg sodium

Nutty Cheese Balls

Prep Time: 20 minutes ★ **Total Time:** 20 minutes + chilling time

These easy-to-make and easy-to-eat snacks are great for a party or can be kept on hand in the refrigerator for a quick snack.

1 **cup pecans or walnuts, toasted**

½ **cup parsley**

½ **cup dried fruit, such as pineapple or a combination of fruits**

3 **scallions**

8 **ounces reduced-fat cream cheese**

2 **cups shredded reduced-fat Cheddar cheese**

½ **teaspoon curry powder**

1. In a food processor, combine the nuts and parsley. Process until the nuts are finely ground. Transfer to a plate.

2. In the food processor, combine the dried fruit and scallions. Pulse until very finely chopped. Add the cream cheese, Cheddar, and curry powder. Process until well combined. Transfer to a small bowl.

3. Divide the mixture evenly in half and shape into 2 large balls, or use a measuring tablespoon to shape into approximately 32 small balls.

4. Gently roll the cheese balls in the nut mixture to lightly coat. Transfer to a serving plate. Cover and refrigerate for at least 2 hours, or up to several days.

Makes 32 servings

Per serving: 65 calories, 3 g protein, 3 g carbohydrates, 5 g total fat, 2 g saturated fat, 0 g fiber, 78 mg sodium

Raspberry-Almond Cheesecake

Prep Time: 15 minutes ★ **Total Time:** 15 minutes

You can use any berry or chopped fresh fruit in this rich, mostly make-ahead dessert.

8 ounces reduced-fat cream cheese, at room temperature

7 ounces 2% plain Greek yogurt

2 tablespoons honey

¼ teaspoon vanilla extract

½ cup graham cracker crumbs

½ pint raspberries

½ cup chopped or sliced almonds, toasted

1. In a medium bowl, with an electric mixer on medium-low speed, beat the cream cheese, yogurt, honey, and vanilla until smooth.

2. Place 2 tablespoons of the crumbs into 4 bowls or tall dessert cups. Top with ⅓ cup of the cream cheese mixture. Divide the raspberries among the cups. Sprinkle with the almonds.

Makes 4 servings

Per serving: 298 calories, 13 g protein, 28 g carbohydrates, 16 g total fat, 7 g saturated fat, 4 g fiber, 346 mg sodium

Strawberry-Banana Crepes

Prep Time: 30 minutes + chilling time ★ **Total Time:** 50 minutes

You can make the entire batch of crepes at once and freeze what you don't use, stacking them with sheets of waxed paper between each, or make as many as you need and store the remaining batter in the refrigerator for a day or two.

½ cup all-purpose flour

¼ cup whole wheat flour

⅛ teaspoon salt

1 cup 1% milk

2 eggs

2 tablespoons + 1 teaspoon light olive oil

2 bananas, thinly sliced (about 2 cups)

1 pound strawberries, sliced (about 4 cups)

½ cup mascarpone cheese

Drizzle

½ cup bittersweet chocolate chips

1. In a medium bowl, whisk together the all-purpose flour, whole wheat flour, and salt. Whisk in the milk, eggs, and 2 tablespoons of the oil. Refrigerate for at least 15 minutes.

2. Heat the remaining 1 teaspoon oil in a small nonstick skillet over medium heat. Brush or swirl the oil so it coats the pan. Pour 2 tablespoons of the batter into the skillet, swirling the batter around so it coats the bottom of the pan.

3. When the top of the crepe appears dry, use a thin spatula to loosen and turn the crepe. Cook for 15 seconds, or until the underside is dry. Use the spatula to transfer the crepe to a plate. Repeat with the remaining batter, stacking the crepes as they are cooked.

4. In a medium bowl, combine the bananas and strawberries. Spread 1 tablespoon of the cheese over half of each crepe. Top each with about ⅓ cup of the fruit and fold the crepe over the filling. Place 1 crepe on each of 8 plates.

5. Place the chocolate chips in a microwaveable bowl and microwave on high power for 1 minute, stirring every 30 seconds, or until melted. Drizzle over the crepes.

Makes 8 servings

Per serving: 260 calories, 6 g protein, 21 g carbohydrates, 19 g total fat, 8 g saturated fat, 4 g fiber, 218 mg sodium

Flourless Chocolate Cake
with Coconut Topping

Prep Time: 15 minutes ★ **Total Time:** 1 hour

Family and friends will never guess the secret ingredient in this light, chocolatey cake that helps keep your blood sugar stable. (Hint: It's a legume.) If you don't like coconut, sprinkle finely chopped nuts over the chocolate topping or leave plain.

Cake

- 1 cup bittersweet chocolate chips
- 1 can (15 ounces) no-salt-added kidney beans, rinsed and drained
- 5 eggs, divided
- ⅓ cup light olive oil
- ¼ cup sugar
- 1 tablespoon vanilla extract
- 1 teaspoon baking powder
- ½ teaspoon baking soda
- ½ teaspoon salt

Topping

- ⅓ cup bittersweet chocolate chips
- ½ teaspoon light olive oil
- ¼ cup unsweetened coconut flakes

1. *To make the cake:* Preheat the oven to 325°F. Lightly coat an 8" × 8" baking pan with cooking spray.

2. Place the chocolate chips in a microwaveable bowl and microwave on high power for 2 to 3 minutes, stirring every minute, or until melted.

3. In a food processor, combine the beans and 2 of the eggs. Process until smooth. Add the oil, sugar, vanilla, baking powder, baking soda, salt, melted chocolate, and the remaining 3 eggs. Process just until blended. Pour into the pan.

4. Bake for 30 minutes, or until a wooden pick inserted in the center of the cake comes out clean. Cool in the pan for 15 minutes. Invert a baking sheet over the pan and carefully turn out the cake. Cool completely. Invert the cake right side up onto a serving plate.

5. *To make the topping:* Place the chocolate chips and oil in a small microwaveable bowl and microwave on high for 1 to 2 minutes, stirring every minute, or until melted. Drizzle over the cake. Top with the coconut. Cut into 12 pieces.

Makes 12 servings

Per serving: 260 calories, 6 g protein, 21 g carbohydrates, 19 g total fat, 8 g saturated fat, 4 g fiber, 218 mg sodium

Orange-Pineapple Ambrosia

Prep Time: 25 minutes ★ **Total Time:** 25 minutes + chilling time

An old-fashioned idea, this fruit salad becomes new again with yogurt replacing the traditional sour cream, and fresh or frozen Bing cherries replacing maraschinos.

½ pineapple, peeled, cored, and cut into bite-size pieces

2 oranges, peeled and cut into sections

1 cup fresh or frozen and thawed pitted Bing cherries, halved

1 cup pecans, toasted and chopped

1 cup shredded unsweetened coconut

½ cup 2% plain Greek yogurt

¼ cup honey

1. In a medium bowl, combine the pineapple, oranges, cherries, pecans, and coconut. Stir in the yogurt and honey.

2. Refrigerate for at least 1 hour or up to 3 hours before serving.

Makes 6 servings

Per serving: 359 calories, 5 g protein, 37 g carbohydrates, 24 g total fat, 10 g saturated fat, 6 g fiber, 11 mg sodium

Roast Pears with Mascarpone Cream

Prep Time: 10 minutes ★ **Total Time:** 40 minutes

You can also try this recipe with fresh peaches, nectarines, or plums.

¼ cup water

2 ripe pears, peeled, cored, and halved lengthwise

2 teaspoons lemon juice

¼ cup no-sugar-added muesli

2 tablespoons honey

¼ cup mascarpone cheese

¼ cup 1% plain Greek yogurt

¼ teaspoon vanilla extract

1. Preheat the oven to 375°F. Bring the water to a boil. Cut a thin sliver from the rounded side of each pear and place in a pie plate. Sprinkle with the lemon juice.

2. Spoon 1 tablespoon of the muesli into each pear half. Drizzle evenly with the honey. Pour the water around the pears.

3. Bake for 30 minutes, basting occasionally with the liquid from the dish and adding another 1 to 2 tablespoons boiling water, if necessary, or until the pears are tender and the topping is crusty.

4. Meanwhile, in a small bowl, stir together the mascarpone, yogurt, and vanilla until well blended.

5. Serve each warm pear half with 2 tablespoons of mascarpone cream.

Makes 4 servings

Per serving: 239 calories, 5 g protein, 28 g carbohydrates, 14 g total fat, 7 g saturated fat, 1 g fiber, 22 mg sodium

Pumpkin Pudding

Prep Time: 10 minutes ★ **Total Time:** 1 hour + chilling time

Just like pumpkin pie, but a little lighter in texture and with nuts on top instead of a crust on the bottom.

1 can (15 ounces) pumpkin

¼ cup sugar

¼ cup honey

3 eggs

1 cup 1% milk

1 teaspoon pumpkin pie spice mix

1 teaspoon vanilla extract

½ cup chopped walnuts

1. Preheat the oven to 325°F. Lightly coat a 1-quart baking dish with cooking spray.

2. In a medium bowl, whisk together the pumpkin, sugar, honey, eggs, milk, spice mix, and vanilla. Pour into the prepared dish.

3. Bake for 45 to 50 minutes, or until the center is just barely set. Remove to a rack. Sprinkle evenly with the walnuts. Cool completely. Refrigerate for at least 2 hours to serve cold.

Makes 8 servings

Per serving: 164 calories, 5 g protein, 22 g carbohydrates, 7 g total fat, 1 g saturated fat, 3 g fiber, 43 mg sodium

Mango-Lime Ice Cream Sundaes

Prep Time: 15 minutes ★ **Total Time:** 15 minutes

You can also use this simple mango sauce as a topping for other desserts, such as plain cake, vanilla pudding, or rice pudding, and even for savory dishes, such as grilled chicken or fish. Look for reduced-fat grated coconut in your supermarket or health food store.

2 ripe mangoes, peeled and pitted

1 tablespoon lime juice

2 tablespoons chopped fresh mint or 1 teaspoon dried, crumbled

2 cups light vanilla ice cream or frozen yogurt

½ cup shredded unsweetened coconut

½ cup chopped pistachios or walnuts

1. In a food processor or blender, combine the mangoes, lime juice, and mint. Process or blend until just slightly chunky.

2. For each sundae, scoop ½ cup of the ice cream or frozen yogurt into a small bowl. Top each with about ¼ cup mango sauce. Sprinkle evenly with the coconut. Top each sundae with 2 tablespoons of the chopped nuts.

Makes 4

Per serving: 337 calories, 8 g protein, 40 g carbohydrates, 18 g total fat, 9 g saturated fat, 5 g fiber, 52 mg sodium

Panna Cotta with Berries

Prep Time: 5 minutes ★ **Total Time:** 25 minutes + chilling time

Panna cotta means "cooked cream" in Italian, but there's no cream in this lightened version. Instead, we used 1% milk and 0% Greek yogurt. Traditionally, these are served unmolded, but there is really no need to do so. They would also look beautiful in wine or martini glasses.

1 cup 1% milk, divided

1½ teaspoons unflavored gelatin

2½ tablespoons sugar

1 tablespoon grated lemon peel

¾ cup 0% plain Greek yogurt

½ teaspoon vanilla extract

¾ cup fresh blueberries, blackberries, or raspberries or a combination

1. Coat four (6-ounce) custard cups or ramekins with cooking spray. Pour ½ cup of the milk into a small bowl. Sprinkle the gelatin over top. Set aside for 5 minutes, or until the gelatin softens.

2. In a small saucepan, using your fingers, rub the sugar and lemon peel together. Stir in the remaining ½ cup milk.

3. Place the saucepan over medium heat and cook, stirring occasionally, for 2 minutes, or until the sugar dissolves and the mixture comes to a simmer. Remove from the heat and whisk in the reserved gelatin mixture. Cover and set aside for 10 minutes.

4. Whisk the yogurt and vanilla into the mixture. Pour into the custard cups and refrigerate for at least 1 hour, or until set.

5. To serve, gently ease the panna cotta away from the edges of the cups, using your fingertips or a small spatula. Invert onto dessert plates, or serve directly from the custard cups. Serve with the berries.

Makes 4 servings

Per serving: 101 calories, 7 g protein, 17 g carbohydrates, 1 g total fat, 0.5 g saturated fat, 1 g fiber, 43 mg sodium

Peaches in Spiced Red Wine

Prep Time: 5 minutes ★ **Total Time:** 1 hour 5 minutes

In the fall and winter, you can use sliced ripe pears instead of peaches. You can also try other nuts to top this dessert. Toasted pine nuts or sliced almonds are especially good.

1 **cup red wine**	1 **tablespoon honey**
¼ **teaspoon ground cinnamon**	2 **ripe peaches, pitted and sliced in wedges**
⅛ **teaspoon ground cardamom (optional)**	3 **tablespoons chopped pistachios**

1. In a small saucepan, bring the wine, cinnamon, and cardamom (if using) to a boil.

2. Remove from the heat and stir in the honey. Add the peaches and let steep at room temperature for at least 1 hour. Transfer to a bowl or jar. Cover and refrigerate for up to 3 days.

3. To serve, spoon the peaches and wine mixture into glasses or dessert bowls. Sprinkle with the pistachios.

Makes 4 servings

Per serving: 129 calories, 2 g protein, 15 g carbohydrates, 3 g total fat, 0.5 g saturated fat, 2 g fiber, 3 mg sodium

Grapefruit and Pomegranate Granita

Prep Time: 10 minutes ★ **Total Time:** 4 hours 10 minutes

Delightfully tart and refreshing, this is the perfect light dessert or intermezzo. To add a little kick, add 1 tablespoon grated ginger to the water and sugar mixture. Let it steep for 15 minutes, then strain and proceed with the recipe.

2 **cups water**	1 **cup 100% pomegranate juice**
2 **tablespoons sugar**	1 **tablespoon lime juice**
1½ **cups 100% grapefruit juice**	8 **sprigs mint (optional)**

1. In a small saucepan, combine the water and sugar and bring to a boil. Stir to dissolve the sugar. Pour into an 8" × 8" baking pan.

2. Add the grapefruit juice, pomegranate juice, and lime juice and stir to mix. Freeze for 4 hours, or until completely frozen.

3. To serve, scrape the surface of the granita with a fork and spoon the scrapings into serving glasses or bowls. (Leftover granita can be frozen for up to 2 months.) Garnish with mint sprigs (if using).

Makes 8 servings

Per serving: 48 calories, 0 g protein, 12 g carbohydrates, 0 g total fat, 0 g saturated fat, 0 g fiber, 10 mg sodium

Part 2

★

Rescue Yourself with Lifestyle

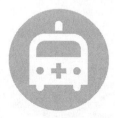

Walk Away from Diabetes in 21 Days!

When I traveled in Cinque Terre, a coastal area of Italy known for its rugged landscape, I was amazed to see people of all ages—carrying beach chairs and coolers—walking up and down steep cliffs with no apparent effort. You'd never see that in America! They were simply used to it.

In other areas near the Mediterranean, I saw families in their Sunday best, without hiking shoes, walking casually along high, steep paths after church. Again, they were just used to it. This kind of everyday walking—nothing fancy—is, I think, part of the reason for the unusually good health of the people there.

If only Americans would adopt this no-big-deal habit. But more than half of us don't get enough physical activity—not even walking—to benefit our health. And yet, if you have diabetes or are at risk for it, walking is one of the easiest, most enjoyable ways to prevent or manage diabetes, protect your heart, and lose weight.

Part of the traditional Mediterranean diet is to get regular physical activity because, as I just illustrated, it's part of the Mediterranean lifestyle. Some scoring plans for adherence to the diet, however, don't measure activity. The Diabetes Rescue Diet does include physical activity because, as you'll see, it's tremendously helpful for both preventing and controlling diabetes.

Not only is walking enjoyable—it works. Study after study shows this. Research links a daily, brisk, 30-minute walk to a reduced diabetes risk of up to 40 percent. It's also been found to cut the risk of death from any and all causes by more than half!

And teamed with a healthy diet, a standing date with a pair of walking shoes can prevent most cases of diabetes in people with impaired glucose tolerance, clinical trials have demonstrated. As a bonus, walking boosts your energy and mood, which makes it far more likely that you'll take better care of your health—which means you'll enjoy a better quality of life.

If you already have diabetes, there's good news for you, too: Lifestyle changes, walking included, are far more effective than some diabetes medications. So if you take an oral diabetes drug, walking just may be a way to reduce your dosage or eliminate it altogether.

The best part of all: Walking requires no special skills; you just get out there and put one foot in front of the other. (You don't even have to walk up cliffs!) This chapter's 21-day program will start you on the path to better health.

Diabetes Takes a Walk

There's no question that anyone can benefit from a daily walk. But walking is an especially smart choice if you have type 2 diabetes or other health problems that keep you from more strenuous activities.

And a brisk 30-minute walk is all you need. Women who walked briskly for at least 30 minutes a day slashed their risk of diabetes by 30 percent, researchers at the Harvard School of Public Health found. Brisk walking is classified as a "moderate intensity" activity. You're walking briskly when you're going faster than usual but not to the point of huffing and puffing, straining, or feeling uncomfortable.

Walking also shrinks dangerous abdominal fat, a known risk factor for diabetes. Excess fat around your abdomen causes inflammation in cells. This swelling makes them even more resistant to insulin,

Walking Tones Your Brain, Too

How about a nice, sharp, youthful brain to go with your healthier heart and better blood sugar? Walking will help your mind stay sharp, too, according to a study of nearly 300 people conducted at the University of Pittsburgh.

The researchers began tracking the physical activity and cognitive (thinking) patterns of the participants (mostly women) in 1989. At the start, all were in good cognitive health and averaged 78 years old. The researchers charted how many blocks each person walked per week.

Nine years later, the participants were given a high-resolution MRI scan to measure brain size. All were "cognitively normal." But 4 years after that, testing showed that a little more than one-third of them had developed mild cognitive impairment or dementia.

By correlating cognitive health, brain scans, and walking patterns, the researchers found that being more physically active appeared to lower the risk of developing memory problems. But more specifically, they concluded that the more you walk, the more gray matter you'll have a decade or more down the road in regions of the brain that are central to thinking. The brain actually shrinks with age, so it's definitely one part of the body you want to keep plump!

Further, the more physically active participants, who had retained more gray matter a decade out, slashed their chances of developing memory problems in half.

the hormone that controls blood sugar, which increases your odds of developing the disease. But women who walked briskly for about an hour a day decreased their belly fat by 20 percent after 14 weeks, a Canadian study found. And they didn't even have to change their eating habits.

Here's another sweet bonus: If you have diabetes, you're more likely to walk off abdominal fat—and your blood sugars will improve as a result of a slimmer belly. In an Australian study, women with diabetes who walked an hour a day, 5 days a week, for 3 months lost belly fat and gained better blood sugar levels—and the benefit to blood sugar was directly related to the loss of belly fat.

In another 4-month study published in *Diabetes Research and Clinical Practice,* researchers in Sweden tested the effects of a walking program—three times a week for 45 to 60 minutes—on people with type 2 diabetes. Compared with a control group that didn't walk, those who did had better blood pressure and cholesterol control and healthier body mass indexes (BMI is a measure of weight in relation to height).

Not only does walking safeguard the health of people with diabetes, it cuts *waaay* back on their health care costs. In a 2008 study, scientists from France randomly assigned 25 people with diabetes to one of two groups—13 were asked to walk twice a week for 30 to 45 minutes, and 12 received their usual treatment. The researchers followed both groups to evaluate their health care costs and exercise effectiveness. At the end of the study, the walking group had slashed their health care costs in half—they cut down on their hospital time and required fewer oral diabetes medications.

Step Up to a Healthier Heart

To keep your heart healthy—an important goal if you have or are at risk of diabetes—walking can't be beat. Several large studies have linked a daily constitutional (as walking used to be called) to a lower risk of cardiovascular disease.

And not just a little lower—up to 40 percent lower for people who walk 30 minutes a day, compared with couch potatoes. Lower blood pressure, better cholesterol numbers, a lower risk of cardiovascular disease . . . you name the heart benefit, and walking probably covers it.

Let's take heart attack, for example. In a study of almost 73,000 women, researchers from Harvard Medical School found that those who walked 3 hours or more per week reduced their risk of a heart attack or other coronary event by 35 percent, compared with women who did not walk.

How Long Do You Have to Walk?

Short answer: not long. From the studies that have been conducted on the link between walking and type 2 diabetes, just 3 hours a week—that's 30 minutes six times a week—confers benefits.

For example, in a 2003 study conducted by the Centers for Disease Control and Prevention (CDC), researchers examined the relationship between walking, as well as other physical activities, with the risk of death in a sample of almost 3,000 people who already had type 2 diabetes. They found that, compared with couch potatoes, those who walked at least 2 hours a week lowered their risk of death by any cause by a not-too-shabby 39 percent and their risk of dying from cardiovascular disease by 34 percent.

However, those who walked 3 to 4 hours a week cut their risk of death from any and all causes by more than half! And that was even when the scientists factored in variables and lifestyle habits that influence the health of people with type 2 diabetes, including age, body mass index, and smoking.

The best part: You don't have to do your whole walk at one time. You can break it up into 10-minute chunks and still reap benefits. That's the conclusion of an 18-month study at the University of Pittsburgh. It found that doing three 10-minute bursts of exercise per day was as beneficial for heart health and weight loss as a single 30-minute workout!

What about people with type 2 diabetes? Does walking also reduce their risk of heart disease? Well, researchers—again from Harvard—looked at the association between walking and the likelihood of cardiovascular events in a group of more than 5,000 women. They found that women with diabetes who got at least 4 hours a week of moderate to vigorous exercise (brisk walking would qualify) had about a 40 percent lower risk of cardiovascular disease and stroke.

Even better, you don't have to huff and puff in order for walking to strengthen your heart. In fact, one study of almost 3,000 people who were tracked by researchers for 8 years found that the protective effects were strongest in people who reported that their walking prompted moderate rather than large increases in their heart and breathing rates.

Walking will also lower your risk of stroke, research suggests. Harvard researchers examined data on the exercise habits of more than 39,000 middle-aged women, tracking them for almost 12 years. Every few years, the women reported how much time they spent on active pursuits, including walking. The women who said they walked 2 or more hours a week reduced their stroke risk by 30 percent.

Walk This Way

There's no easier workout than walking. But most walkers aren't aware that they might be walking inefficiently and making it harder on themselves. Maybe you jolt and jerk when you walk, for example, or swing your arms too much. Such offenses might sound minor, but over time, their effects can mount and put you down with a walking injury.

Here's the rundown on how to correct some of the most common mistakes walkers make. Don't take another step until you've checked these out!

Watch your posture. Whether you walk bent over with your head down or do the opposite, leaning back when you walk, you're setting yourself up for injury. Leaning too far forward or backward throws your body off balance, putting undue stress on your lower back. The result? Strain and pain.

To straighten up, hold your head high, so your neck and the rest of your spine form a straight line. Don't tuck your chin into your neck, and look well ahead of you. (Experts' advice on the distance ranges from 10 to 30 feet ahead.) Also, make sure your shoulders are relaxed and your stomach is tucked. A way to check yourself is to take a big breath every 5 minutes and exhale strongly. Notice how your shoulders drop? That's how you want to carry yourself.

Keep your arms down. Flapping arms can not only slow you down but also set you up for injuries such as shin splints. By all means, allow your arms to swing back and forth when you walk, but don't let them flap willy-nilly from side to side. Instead, keep your arms bent

90 degrees, and place your elbows close to your sides, so they drive back, not outward.

Tread softly. Are you a clomper or a stomper? If so, you need to lighten up—softening your footfall will save your feet and legs. When you step forward, let your heel strike the ground gently before your foot rolls forward, then push off from your toes.

Treat yourself to a pedometer. These little gadgets count how many steps you take—and you walk more when you clip one to your waistband. In a review article published in the *Journal of the American Medical Association*, Stanford University researchers examined the medical literature on the effectiveness of pedometers. In their review, which included almost 3,000 people, they found that walking with a pedometer increased study participants' overall physical activity by 27 percent.

The increase in physical activity had other benefits—it lowered blood pressure, risk of stroke, and weight, the team found. You can pick up a pedometer at your local big-box store for less than 10 bucks—not a bad investment, I'd say. (You can also use it to count the number of steps you take during the course of your day. See "Step It Up Throughout Your Day" on page 268 for easy ways to step up your step count.)

If you don't use a pedometer, use your wristwatch to count the number of minutes you walk on our program. Your schedule is all laid out for you ahead.

Walking with Diabetes

Ready to walk toward better health? Great—just talk with your doctor or health care team first. Typically, people with diabetes can start a walking program without having any tests, but it's best to follow your doctor's recommendations. Once you get the green light, these tips can help ensure that your walks are safe and enjoyable.

Before you walk, talk. I just said this, but it bears repeating: If you're new to this walking thing, give your doctor or diabetes care team a call. Ask how much walking you can do each day and if you should adjust your medications or insulin, depending on the intensity, duration, or time of day of your exercise. Your doctor can also review the

Try a Little Togetherness

Some people like to walk in solitude to enjoy nature and be alone with their thoughts. But if it's hard for you to get started, you might want to join a walking group, especially if you take medication for diabetes.

To evaluate whether group walks would benefit the health of people with type 2 diabetes, researchers in Italy split 59 people with diabetes into two groups. The first group got the standard recommendation to make lifestyle changes and was encouraged to walk. The second group, however, actually walked—three times a week for 45 minutes, supervised by a trainer. The team tested everyone's A1c and overall physical activity, and monitored their diabetes medications.

After 4 months, the walking group was in better physical shape. Also, compared with the nonwalking group, the walkers' fasting glucose and total cholesterol numbers were better. But best of all, 33 percent of them were able to reduce their medication—or eliminate it altogether—compared with only 5 percent of the nonwalking group!

To find a walking group near you, do an Internet search, plugging in your town or zip code and the phrase "walking group." Or simply ask a friend to join you. You'll walk off weight—and diabetes risk—together!

latest readings on your cholesterol, A1c, and lipids before you start your program, so you can compare the "before" and "after" numbers.

Treat your feet right. When you have diabetes, wounds heal more slowly, especially on the feet, so it's critical to take care of your feet and prevent blisters. Walk in good shoes that fit properly. I recommend buying your walking shoes at an athletic-shoe store, where employees are trained to fit shoes. Wear good socks, too, made of a fabric such as Coolmax, which helps wick away sweat and prevent blisters.

Keep on top of your blood sugar level. Before and after your walk, check your blood sugar. If it's too low or high, postpone your walk.

Drink up! Before and after you walk, drink a big glass of water. Sip during activity, too.

Pack a snack. Be prepared in case you or your walking partner detects signs of low blood sugar. After your walk, you may need to eat more carbohydrates than usual to prevent delayed hypoglycemia.

Wear ID. Wear a medical identification bracelet or necklace that says you have diabetes—just in case.

Walk Away from Diabetes Dangers in 21 Days

If you have diabetes, you can't walk away from it—but you can walk away from its dangerous complications. This walking workout will boost your energy, rev your metabolism, and benefit your blood sugar and cardiovascular health. You might even drop some weight! You don't have to wait long for results, either—all these benefits can be yours in just 21 days or less!

You'll get the best results if you walk briskly, just slightly out of your comfort zone. Let me be clear: *your* comfort zone. No need to go at a racewalker's pace to reap the rewards of this program. But because you'll be walking in a variety of ways—long walks and short, higher-intensity bouts and one nice, comfortable stroll per week—you'll keep your metabolism guessing, which cranks up your calorie burn.

Your 21-Day Walking Schedule

Here's a suggested schedule, with a daily tip that can make your walking easier, more comfortable, or simply more fun. Start and finish each workout with 5 minutes of slow walking to warm up and cool down your muscles. On Sunday, simply enjoy your walk—you've earned it.

First things first: Walk safe! Canvass the area at the time of day you plan to be out walking. If your path takes you along the road, don't walk on the shoulder. Better yet, find a park. If you're unfamiliar with the route, drive it looking for danger zones—unleashed dogs in yards, for example. And after each and every walk, check your feet for injuries.

Day 1: Walk 10 minutes.

Today's tip: Soak up your surroundings. Notice the sky, clouds, and flowers. Say hi to your neighbors. Keep your eyes focused several feet in front of you so that you can anticipate terrain and traffic.

Day 2: Walk 10 minutes.

Today's tip: Goals are a great way to get motivated to exercise. Write down your goal and place it where you can look at it often. Make your goal realistic and achievable. Modify it as you go along, making it more challenging. If you feel your exercise motivation deteriorating, take a look at your goal.

Day 3: Walk 12 minutes.

Today's tip: Did you get those new walking shoes? Wear well-cushioned walking shoes, a hat with a protective visor, and sunscreen. Choose sweat-wicking clothes to keep you dry.

Day 4: Walk 12 minutes.

Today's tip: If you're using a pedometer, clip it on properly. Incorrect placement may result in only a portion of your steps being counted until you reposition it. To count steps accurately, a pedometer must hang vertically from your waist, aligned over your knee. Clip it to the tiny pocket just below the waistband of your jeans and you'll know it's in the right place.

Day 5: Walk 13 minutes.

Today's tip: Feeling a little sore? As a walking newbie, you may be taking longer strides and using more of your lower leg muscles on uneven surfaces and for push-off. To avoid injury and muscle soreness, walk at a slower pace for 5 minutes before your workout.

Day 6: Walk 13 minutes.

Today's tip: Buy or borrow an MP3 player and pump up your walk with your favorite tunes—the ones that never fail to boost your mood and rev you up. A study from Ghent University in Belgium proves that the right tempo pushes you to speed up, so you work off calories faster. I like rollicking Irish reels and hornpipes, but I also love up-tempo Neil Diamond songs like "Solitary Man," "America," and "Sweet Caroline"—perfect for spirited walking. Whatever turns your motor on!

Day 7: Walk 15 minutes.

Today's tip: Celebrate little successes—like the fact that you're done with your first full week of walking. Pay attention to your energy levels, how you're sleeping, and how your clothes fit. You should notice some improvements in as little as 2 weeks, though the scale may take a bit longer to reflect how well you're doing.

Total for Week 1: 85 minutes

Week 2: Getting into the Swing

Day 8: Walk 15 minutes.

Today's tip: There is no bigger motivator than seeing results. Track your progress so you can look back and see how well you've done. Let others know that you are exercising, and brag about the progress you have made. Your friends and family can be your support system to keep you motivated.

Day 9: Walk 15 minutes.

Today's tip: If you like the feedback that treadmills give about pace and distance, try timing yourself on an outdoor walking track. Most tracks are ¼ mile. If you walk four laps in 15 minutes, your pace is 4 miles per hour.

Day 10: Walk 17 minutes.

Today's tip: Feel like lounging on the couch instead of lacing up your walking shoes? A simple affirmation such as "I can do it!" repeated over and over, or simply stating out loud your personal reasons for walking, can get you out the door.

Day 11: Walk 17 minutes.

Today's tip: Create an exercise "menu." Get to know your rhythms and have a walking plan for each mood. Feeling fatigued? Head for your most relaxing, most naturally beautiful route. Keyed up from work? Walk a bit more briskly—crank it up and burn off that nervous energy!

Day 12: Walk 18 minutes.

Today's tip: Use visualization daily. Picture yourself completing your walk—easily, enjoyably, almost effortlessly. Use your senses to make the visualization as vivid as possible. See the sun shining, hear the birds chirping around you, feel the leaves or gravel crunching under your feet as you stride with confidence. Believe in yourself: You *can* do this!

Day 13: Walk 18 minutes.

Today's tip: Don't have a dog or a toddler? Borrow one for your walk! There's nothing like chasing after a 3-year-old to keep you moving at a brisk pace without even realizing it!

Day 14: Walk 20 minutes.

Today's tip: You're two-thirds through our program! Instead of saving personal rewards for distant, huge goals, like a 20-pound weight loss, make them behavior oriented. Set a goal to finish out this program, and at the end of Day 21's walk, treat yourself to a nonfood reward, like a couple of new songs for your walking playlist or a new pair of walking shorts.

Total for Week 2: 120 minutes

Week 3: Heading into the Homestretch

Day 15: Walk 20 minutes.

Today's tip: Revisit your goal from Day 2. Keeping up with your walking program can sometimes be as simple as reminding yourself why you got started in the first place. How are your blood sugar numbers these days? Are you more able to keep up with your grand-kids or your demanding schedule? Is your waistband a little looser? Think about your goal and how your walking routine is helping you achieve it.

Day 16: Walk 23 minutes.

Today's tip: Who—or what—truly inspires you? Find a photo and put it where you'll see it every day. Maybe it's a shot of you and your spouse on vacation, looking trim and fit. Or you looking good in size 10 jeans. Or a photo of Lance Armstrong, who overcame so much to

---

Tips from a (Might as Well Be) Professional Walker

At one point in my life, I was practically a professional walker. I wrote books on walking, started a national walking club that had tens of thousands of members, and even had walking rallies in various walker-friendly cities. I also worked with the President's Council on Physical Fitness to develop special awards for walking.

I currently walk nearly every day, and I find it's not only good for my health but also for controlling my weight and clearing my head. We purposely vacation at a resort area that has miles of walking trails and a long beach where my wife and I and our dog, Seamus, go for long walks and watch for dolphins. Here are some of my personal tips, based on many years of wearing out walking shoes.

- Many walking shoes are too much like running shoes, with thick heels and a heavy structure to reduce shock. But walking has much less impact on your joints than running. So when you're ready for your next pair of shoes, try on one of the new lighter styles that are now on the market. When I asked my shoe seller (trained to fit shoes) for a lighter, more flexible pair, he brought out the Saucony Kinvara, which I took for a test spin outside and loved. Each shoe weighs only 8 ounces, has a lower heel than other shoes, and generally is perfect for walking or racewalking, which I do sometimes.

---

become a champion athlete. Look at that photo every day when you wake up and before you go to sleep. This act will help you reconnect with the reasons exercising is important to you—and set you up for success tomorrow.

Day 17: Walk 25 minutes.

Today's tip: Add more movement to your day! Now that you've got this walking thing down, branch out and add more activity. See page 268 for some easy ways to fit more movement into your day, beyond your daily walk.

- Shop for your shoes at the end of the day. That's when your feet are largest. If you walk in the morning, you can always make small adjustments in size with socks. Wear your walking socks when shopping, too. Some styles are really thick, and you may need to go half a size larger with your shoes to accommodate them.

- Walk at a pace that's comfortable for you. If you want to try increasing your pace—even for half a minute or so—don't do it by extending your stride. Instead, take shorter strides, but walk a little faster. If you have a digital watch, count your steps for 30 seconds or a minute, and then try increasing that number by just two steps. When that gets easy, go for another extra step or two.

- If you have diabetes, always wear a belt pack with some blood sugar boosters like glucose tablets in case your blood sugar unexpectedly begins to plummet.

- If you're not in the best of health, walk with a partner.

- Keep a walking log—either your own or the one on page 270. Seeing how far you've come—and setting new challenges for yourself—will encourage you to keep walking.

Day 18: Walk 27 minutes.

Today's tip: Whatever your reasons for walking, if you don't keep them right in your face, you may not make it out the door! Do whatever it takes to keep yourself going: Ask a friend to walk with you. Post your reasons for walking all over—on the bathroom mirror, the refrigerator door, your computer monitor at work, or even the dashboard of your car—wherever you will see them throughout the day. Write your workout into your schedule—and set reminders so that you'll be ready to head outside or onto the treadmill when your alarm dings. And ask your spouse for support, even if that means he or she will push you out the door!

Walk Away from Stress

Reducing the impact of stress is a good way to reduce the impact of diabetes. People with type 2 diabetes who attended just five stress-management sessions run by Duke University Medical Center lowered their A1c blood sugar—the gold standard for measuring long-term glucose control—by a significant amount.

Similar good results in a small group of people with diabetes were seen in a much more involved program based on the work of Jon Kabat-Zinn, PhD. That program, called mindfulness-based stress reduction, is an intense 8-week affair, but what caught my attention was a component called mindful walking. I believe that any kind of walking reduces stress, but if you can boost the effect, why not go for it?

After I looked into mindful walking, also called a walking meditation, I realized I'd been doing it for years—or, at least, a variation of it. Most versions emphasize very slow walking, which doesn't do much for your cardio fitness. I like to walk briskly, as briskly as I can. So I adapted it for use at any walking pace—whatever's comfortable for you. Here's my own version of a stress-reducing, soul-cleansing walk.

1. When you begin your walk, act and feel as though you are the happiest person in the world. I got this beautiful idea from the Buddhist monk and

---

Day 19: Walk 27 minutes.

Today's tip: If you haven't been charting your progress, now's the time to begin. It'll keep you walking beyond our 21-day program. Use whatever you wish—the walking log on page 270, a high-tech online tracker, or an old-fashioned fitness journal—but give it a try. Are you walking for longer durations? Feeling less achy? Do you have more energy and focus afterward? Are you more optimistic or in a better mood when you return? Seeing improvements will send your motivation sky-high. These are all great observations to make as you continue walking regularly.

author Thich Nhat Hanh. If you can do that, he says, you have succeeded at a walking meditation.

2. Pay close attention to everything you see and feel in the present moment: your breathing, the rhythm of your legs, the trees, the sky, the breeze or mist or sun on your face. Don't think about these things; just feel them.

3. When something that is not in the present slips into your mind—what happened before or what may happen in the future—politely remove it. There's plenty of time for it later in the day.

4. To help yourself stay in the present, notice little things you're doing. Check your posture: Are you standing straight, with your shoulders loose, not bunched up? Are you dragging your heels? Don't lecture yourself; just make a correction. If you have a digital watch, you may want to keep track of your steps per minute. The idea is not to increase them, just notice them. It's fun to see if you can keep the strides the same, minute after minute. This isn't thinking; it's just being aware of the present.

5. Try saying positive things to yourself in rhythm with your steps. Every step is health. Every step is peace. Thank you for this beautiful day!

Day 20: Walk 28 minutes.

Today's tip: To keep you in the walking habit, invite a friend. Lots of people walk in pairs or even threesomes every day. Conversation always beats boredom. Just make sure you're maintaining the pace you want, as talking can slow you down.

Day 21: Walk 30 minutes.

Today's tip: Congratulations—you hit the 30-minute milestone! Don't rest on your laurels, though. Day 22 and beyond beckon. Keeping up with your program is up to you now, but you've got a solid foundation that, if you follow it faithfully, will keep you healthy and vital for the rest of your life.

Total for Week 3: 180 minutes

Step It Up Throughout Your Day

Team the walking program with this 10-step guide to taking more steps. Here are some easy ways to add steps to your day, apart from your daily walk.

1. If you live or work in an area with shops nearby, park your car and commit to using it only to reach destinations more than a mile from your home or office.

2. If you drive to work, park a distance from your office and walk the rest of the way.

3. Park farther away from your destination—the supermarket, bank, school, work. At the mall, park at the opposite end of the store you'll visit. In apartment complexes, park the car and retrieve the mail from the central mail bay on foot.

4. At work, use the stairs instead of the elevator.

5. Pace or walk in place while on the phone, especially during long conversations or conference calls.

6. Frequent venues (farmers' markets, museums, art galleries, parks, sporting events) and choose activities (hiking, yard work,

shopping, kite flying) that require walking. Discover and patronize local neighborhood businesses that are easily reached on foot.

7. When you go to the supermarket, shop in a zigzag pattern. For example, from the dairy aisle, walk six aisles down to pick up laundry detergent. Then go to the bread aisle (usually next to the dairy area), then go to the opposite side of the supermarket to the produce aisle. You get the idea. (Do write out a list so you won't forget anything!) You'll make several trips back and forth across the store, but it is a great way to add movement to your day.

8. This tip is for city folks: If you typically approach a street corner, see no traffic, and start crossing before reaching the exact corner, you're cutting a handful of steps off your trip with each corner. Instead, walk to the corner anyway. Or if you come to a stoplight and aren't in a hurry, cross the street, and then cross back at a red light farther down. It doesn't add a lot of extra time to your trip, but it's more steps.

9. Hide the TV remote. Remember when there were no remotes? Sure you do. Put yours away for the duration of the program. If you must use the remote to change channels, get up from the couch and take it right up to the TV.

10. During commercials, get up and walk around the house. If you typically watch 2 or 3 hours of television a night, you could add countless extra steps during each 2-minute commercial break!

Your 21-Day Walking Log

Now that you've got a walking plan in place, you might find it helpful to track your walks. On the following page, we've provided a table where you can log your activity for each day on the plan. To keep logging after the first 3 weeks, photocopy our chart or create your own!

Log Your Walks!

You don't have to use a walking log, but recording the number of steps you take and time you spend walking over the next 3 weeks—and beyond—will help you track your progress over time. Six months or a year from now, you can look back at Day 1 and marvel at how far you've come!

DAY	MINUTES	COMMENTS/NOTES
1		
2		
3		
4		
5		
6		
7		
8		
9		
10		
11		
12		
13		
14		
15		
16		
17		
18		
19		
20		
21		

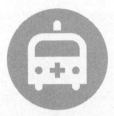

Gardening to the Rescue!

My wife is the gardener in our family, and since it's May as I write this, I asked her what she's put in this year. This is her list.

- ★ Salad greens (three kinds!)
- ★ Spinach
- ★ Sugar snap peas
- ★ String beans
- ★ Tomatoes (beefsteaks for salads and sandwiches; Romas to can)
- ★ Carrots
- ★ Zucchini
- ★ Radishes
- ★ Potatoes (picked small, they melt in your mouth)

That's in her raised bed garden (totally organic, by the way). She also has a "kitchen garden" near the patio, where she grows various herbs, cherry tomatoes, and jalapeño peppers.

If you have or are concerned about diabetes, gardening may the

271

single healthiest activity you can engage in, for a couple of reasons. First, when you grow veggies—either a few or a gardenful—you typically eat what you coax out of the dirt. You can walk by veggies at the supermarket, but you're not going to let your own sugar snap peas wilt on the vine, *are* you? And in fact, a number of studies have found that diabetes rates are lower in areas with community gardens or places where backyard gardening is more common.

Second, everything you grow in your garden is allowed on the Diabetes Rescue Diet. Everything! You can't say that about any supermarket or Whole Foods store or even a farmers' market. There's always someone selling doughnuts!

Finally, as you'll see in a moment, to tend a vegetable garden is to exercise. However, most people who garden—wrapped up in the enjoyment of digging, planting, and harvesting—don't even realize they're working up a decent sweat!

But on the Diabetes Rescue Diet, gardening is for pleasure—a healthy activity that's also good for the soul. So consider planting a garden this year, even if it's just a few pots of patio tomatoes. This chapter can help you get started. No matter what you plant, every bite benefits your health.

"Exercise" That Grows on You

One of the primary components of managing diabetes is getting enough physical exercise. Active gardeners easily get more than the recommended 150 minutes per week, and those who garden just for fun get slightly less than that, according to research from Kansas State University.

No problem, if you follow our walking program (see Walk Away from Diabetes in 21 Days! on page 252). Gardening fits right in with our recommendation to put more movement into your everyday life. A little or a lot, every extra minute counts!

Another great thing about gardening: Depending on the activity, it's not quite as hard on your body as, say, jogging and other types of moderate to strenuous exercise. This means that regardless of your

Grow Veggies—And Satisfaction, Too!

It's hard not to enjoy life when you're surrounded by flowers and vegetables and all the wildlife they attract—and now there's science to confirm that gardening really does lift your mood. Professors from the University of Texas and Texas A&M asked 298 older adults how they would rate their "zest for life," levels of optimism, and overall resolution and fortitude. They found that gardeners had significantly higher scores in all those areas than nongardeners.

Considering that antidepressant use among adults over 65 has nearly tripled since the 1980s, gardening could be as useful as Prozac for warding off the blues.

age, you can always enjoy puttering in the garden. There are a lot of activities with a wide range of physical exertion levels you can do in your garden, so you're bound to find the level that feels right to you.

And although the Diabetes Rescue Diet isn't about losing weight, it doesn't hurt that you can burn 100 to 120 calories in 30 minutes of light gardening, such as weeding by hand, and more when you dig and rake.

And yes, gardening really does benefit your health. According to a report in the *Journal of Applied Physiology,* studies suggest that physically active people have a 30 to 50 percent lower risk of developing type 2 diabetes, compared with sofa spuds. A similar lower risk is seen for coronary heart disease, the report says—a major threat to anyone but especially someone who has diabetes.

I love the fact that a simple, natural activity like gardening can help cut your risk of major health problems smack in half. What's more, the authors say, risk is reduced with as little as 30 minutes of physical activity a day. No need to get sunstroke out there!

Still, in that half hour, challenge yourself to move whenever you can. For instance, instead of setting out the sprinkler to water your garden, stand and water it with the hose. You might also pull weeds by hand, at least for a few minutes.

For Perfect Peace, Play in the Dirt

One of the least-appreciated risk factors for diabetes is stress. And it's not minor! For 15 years, an unusual study in England followed nearly 6,000 middle-aged men and women whose work-related stress levels were periodically checked.

Women with high stress levels, the researchers found, were nearly twice as likely to develop type 2 diabetes over those 15 years. Other studies have revealed much the same thing: more stress = more diabetes.

Experience has taught many gardeners that their time tilling the soil does in fact reduce stress. But that's just a feeling. Is there any scientific proof?

A 2011 report in the *Journal of Health Psychology* describes an experiment designed to test that very notion. First, the researchers took a group of people and subjected them all to a standard stress-inducing experience. Then they randomly assigned half the group

---

Keep Your Feet Garden-Safe

Gardening is a great activity if you have diabetes. Just make sure to practice good foot care.

For example, wear the right shoes. Gardening clogs or sandals could subject your unexposed skin to injury by the poke of a twig, perhaps, or a sharp stone. Always inspect your feet after gardening (or simply every day). If you see a puncture or scrape, wash it with soap and water, apply an antibiotic ointment and a Band-Aid, and call your podiatrist to ask if you should come in. Then keep an eye on the wound for a week or so to monitor for any delayed infection.

Don't wear old, worn shoes, either. They're too soft and bend too easily. And because the foot joints of people with diabetes are more likely to sustain damage when the feet are subjected to extended stress, it's important to wear shoes with stiffer soles. Or garden in a kneeling or seated position, reducing your body weight over the balls of your feet.

---

to 30 minutes of outdoor gardening and the other half to reading a book indoors. While all this was going on, the researchers measured their levels of cortisol—a stress hormone—and gave them verbal tests as well.

Both groups were less stressed after the experiment was over, but the gardeners significantly more so. And "positive mood" was fully restored in the gardeners, while it actually grew worse in the readers!

We have to congratulate these scientists for what they call "the first experimental evidence that gardening can promote relief from acute stress." You knew it all along, you say? But did you know it's better than curling up with a book?

Perfect nutrition. Lower risk of diabetes because of physical activity. Lower risk of diabetes from stress reduction. The satisfaction of picking salad greens, cukes, and bell peppers still warm from the sun.

It's hard to beat that—all from one simple, fun activity! If you have access to a patch of soil, make gardening part of your Diabetes Rescue Diet.

Gardening: Many Ways to Grow

Maybe you've always wanted to garden but never quite knew where to start. Here's how.

Your basic backyard veggie patch. According to my friends at *Organic Gardening* magazine, gardening is not hard. Yes, growing a veggie patch takes time and attention. But if you have access to sunshine and water, you can do it.

The best way to learn is by doing, but it doesn't hurt to read up on the subject. My pals have put together a beginners' guide that touches on the basics of organic gardening and the keys to success they've learned over the years. They offer a wealth of advice on how to get started. To access the guide, log on to the *Organic Gardening* Web site: www.organicgardening.com/learn-and-grow.

If you decide to do an outdoor veggie garden, invite your kids or grandkids to grab a spade, rake, or hoe and get dirty with you. Evidence shows that parents who garden are more likely to pass this knowledge on to their children and thus can begin to break cycles of

Raised Beds: The Easy Way to Grow

Having a very productive garden is much easier than you might think. The secret is to use raised garden beds, which can be built literally anywhere, including on a small spot of grass on your lawn.

You don't need to dig up the ground, as you would with an ordinary garden. You can place your raised bed right on top of the grass, which will die and turn into compost, helping to nourish your plants. And you don't have to build anything yourself, either. Ready-to-use raised bed kits are sold at big-box stores like Home Depot, large garden-supply stores, and online.

The size is up to you—4 feet by 4 feet might be good for starters. Install the sides, then fill it up with a mixture of dirt or potting soil and a good helping of compost—all of which can be bought at any garden shop. Be sure to place your beds in a spot where they'll get good sun. Plant your seeds or already-started plants, water them regularly, and watch them grow.

Maybe the best thing about raised bed gardening is that if you plant the vegetables close together, weeding will be reduced close to 90 percent, compared with what the usual garden requires. I cover my beds with black plastic weighted down with bricks in late fall, so they're still weed free in springtime.

An excellent guide is *Square Foot Gardening* (Rodale, 2005) by Mel Bartholomew. He even shows you how to have a garden that produces nearly year-round.

---

diabetes. That's as welcome a gift as a paper bag full of homegrown zucchini!

Container gardening. Never even had a houseplant? Test the gardening waters: Try growing a tomato or pepper plant in a pot or two in your yard—or windowsill, patio, balcony, or doorstep. All of these small spaces provide sufficient room for a productive mini garden. For a very small investment of time and money, you will have the satisfaction of plucking a ripe tomato off the vine and deciding if gardening is for you. Almost any vegetable that will grow in a typical backyard garden will also do well as a container-grown plant, including tomatoes, peppers, eggplant, beans, lettuce, and squash.

Community gardens. If you live in a city or want to try gardening before digging up your yard, this is a great option. To find a community garden in your area, call your county cooperative extension. The number's listed in your phone book. Or try a neighborhood association, local nursery, the mayor's office, or the town's garden club. You're sure to pick up tons of tips and techniques from the gardener a few plots down from you.

The Herb Garden:
Small Commitment, Big Flavor

If you don't want to commit to a veggie patch, consider an herb garden—either a tiny outdoor patch or a collection of pots indoors. Fresh herbs do so much to perk up even the simplest meals, and they're an easy way to add authentic Mediterranean flavor to the Diabetes Rescue Diet. Wouldn't it be nice to step outside your kitchen door or out on your balcony and pluck some fresh basil and oregano?

If you have a backyard, you might try your hand at a tiny outdoor plot. If you want an indoor herb garden, you can grow your plants in a variety of containers, from flowerpots to tin wash bins and watering troughs. Just make sure there are holes in the bottom to allow water out—herbs need proper drainage. You can find out the how-tos at the *Organic Gardening* Web site: www.organicgardening.com.

If you're an herb newbie, you may be wondering what varieties to grow. You might start with herbs commonly used in Mediterranean cuisine, including basil, oregano, and rosemary. Other common cooking herbs include cilantro, parsley, sage, and thyme.

My wife tells me that herbs are easy to grow if you meet their basic requirements. Most herbs do best in full to part sun—about 6 to 8 hours of sun a day—and thrive in any good garden soil, as long as it drains well when you water it. Once you get them in the ground or in pots, you don't have to do much. Sun and water (a good watering twice a week is all that's needed) are enough. When you're ready to use your herbs, snip off the top leaves, which encourages the plant to grow.

Once you grow your herbs, it's time to use them. This mini cheat sheet can help you pair your herbs with the right dishes. As you can see, you can add them to plenty of Mediterranean-style dishes.

★ Oregano with vegetables or pasta
★ Sage with cooked beans, fish, or chicken (sprinkle on pizza, too!)
★ Sweet basil with chicken or fish, pasta, and tomatoes
★ Mint with tabbouleh or fruit salad
★ Rosemary with chicken or new potatoes
★ Dill with chicken or fish
★ Tarragon with fish, chicken, or salads
★ Thyme with poultry, fish, vegetables, or salads
★ Cilantro with pasta, salads, fish, or salsas

Take the Ache Out of Gardening

Maybe you've grown an outdoor vegetable garden for years and love it. What you don't love is the achiness that comes with standing, stooping, leaning, kneeling, and crouching—especially if you aren't as young and limber as you used to be. (Who is?)

But you don't have to give up the pleasures of homegrown tomatoes or fresh-picked greens. These tips from the pros at Chicago Botanic Garden can help you experience the pleasure of gardening rather than the pain. While these suggestions may seem obvious, most of us don't practice them until *after* we can't stand upright. So don't just know them—practice them!

Set attainable goals. When it comes to gardening, slow and steady is best. Unless you're planting an indoor herb garden, don't plan to plant an entire vegetable patch on a Sunday afternoon. If you do, you'll wind up sore and exhausted. Set modest goals, and assess your progress and how you feel every couple of hours.

Pace yourself. You will work longer and stronger if you go at a task steadily than if you push to finish a big project.

Take breaks. Every hour, give yourself 5 minutes to stretch, sit down, and drink to replenish the fluids lost from your exertion. You'll more than compensate for those idle 5 minutes with increased productivity during the other 55 minutes of the hour. Place chairs in the shade around your garden so you are reminded to relax in them.

Beware of bending and reaching. You are most vulnerable to injury when you are bending at the waist and reaching. You're also more prone to losing your balance and falling in this position. If you must bend, do so with your knees rather than your back. And position yourself close enough to your task so that you are not reaching. Even pulling weeds puts more strain on your lower back than you realize.

Ask for help. This may be the toughest advice to take when you are determined to make it through your list of chores. But if you have a heavy or awkwardly balanced object to move, get assistance from a friend or neighbor. Whether you are lifting something alone or with help, hold it at your side or close to your body in front to avoid back strain.

Have fun! Your garden doesn't have to look like the ones you see on the home and garden channel on TV. Whether it's a few pots near a sunny window or a full-on veggie patch, your garden will grow *you* as much as you grow *it*. There's a saying that gardening is a labor of love—a treadmill is just labor. Take that to heart, and enjoy your time in the sun!

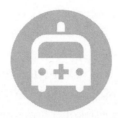

The Rescue Eating-Out Guide

We love to eat out—from fast-food burgers and chicken to nouvelle cuisine, from chain restaurants to the Chinese place on the corner. Unfortunately, when it comes to our health, there's strong evidence to suggest that our passion for dining out is doing us in.

Sometimes you know what you're getting into—say, when you order a fat or sugar bomb like a Monster Thickburger at Hardee's (1,290 calories) or the Triple Chocolate Meltdown at Applebee's (820 calories). But it's also possible to order what sounds like a healthy meal and get ambushed.

Here's one example: the Pecan-Crusted Chicken Salad at Applebee's. It sounds healthy, and pecans and chicken are healthy foods. But the regular portion packs an incredible 1,360 calories and 80 grams of fat, 17 of them saturated. If you control your carbs, you could really be fooled. While pecans and chicken contain virtually no carbs, this salad packs 117 grams of them, according to Applebee's online nutrition information.

How could a meal that sounds so good for you go so wrong? Let's break it down.

It's not that this dish doesn't contain healthy ingredients (romaine lettuce, mandarin oranges, celery, pecans, chicken). It's that it contains entirely too much of them, as well as less-healthy items. In other words, the portion size is huge, which is typical of restaurant meals. Studies have found that most portions at any restaurant are two to eight times larger than the servings defined by the USDA.

So by virtue of size alone, this salad contains a lot of calories, many of which are high in carbs (mandarin oranges, sweet-glazed pecans, dried cranberries) and saturated fat (blue cheese crumbles, full-fat dressing). I don't know how much honey balsamic vinaigrette the chain adds, but I do know from the nutritional information that if you order the very same salad without dressing, you'll save 460 calories.

But you want this salad? You can have it. Just perform a daring Rescue.

Order the half portion without dressing (600 calories).

Hold the glazed pecans and cranberries—you'll ease down the carb count.

Either enjoy the flavorful blue cheese crumbles as "dressing" or hold the crumbles and request a low-fat dressing on the side.

Three simple Rescues and you slice off a major portion of calories, unhealthy fats, and carbohydrates.

The bottom line: If you have diabetes, you can learn to Rescue restaurant meals like the one above (and trust me, you'll have to). The happy truth is that you can dine out anywhere if you become an educated foodie. This isn't hard to do. The simple strategy and practical tips in this chapter will help you evade the traps, make smart choices, and enjoy a tasty, healthy restaurant meal anytime, anywhere.

10 Ways to Rescue Any Restaurant Meal, Anytime

We'll get to specific types of restaurants in a moment. The tips that follow lay the groundwork for a healthy meal anywhere, anytime. Use as many as possible and you'll start to rescue your meal even before you place your napkin on your lap.

1. **"Order" before you go.** Virtually all national chain restaurants have Web sites, where they post the nutrition profile of every item on their menus. Some of them even let you build and customize a meal. If you know you'll be dining at a particular chain, go online and choose your meal based on the nutrition information. (Just type the name of the restaurant followed by "nutrition" into your browser.) This strategy allows you to enjoy a healthy, tasty meal without guilt, gluttony, or glucose explosions. When you order before you go, you don't have to guess what's healthy—you know. And learning that the appetizer or entrée you wanted packs 1,200 calories tends to take care of temptation real quick.

2. **Think "eat," not "treat."** We eat too many meals outside our homes to consider each one a treat. So whenever you dine out, eat normally all day *and* order a healthful restaurant meal. (Watch those portion sizes, too.) This is a smarter, healthier strategy than skipping breakfast and lunch to "spend" those calories on a blowout meal or going out for a huge breakfast or lunch and starving yourself the rest of the day.

3. **Order Diabetes Rescue style.** If you're at a restaurant where you can order grilled fish or lean meat, a portion of whole grains or legumes, and veggies with a drizzle of olive oil, you can't go wrong. More eateries than you might think can accommodate this menu. Add one glass of wine (if you drink) or fruit for dessert. Delicious!

4. **Water down your appetite.** Ask for water with lemon and drink two glasses, if possible, before your food arrives. This has been shown to cut down calorie consumption in a major way.

5. **Have a loose interpretation of "menu."** A menu is a flexible document. Treat it that way. Don't be afraid to ask for the breakfast fruit cup for dessert or request a skewer of grilled shrimp, which usually tops a dinner salad, as an appetizer. Or skip the dinner entrée altogether and combine a salad with a low-fat appetizer.

A Daring Rescue at Starbucks

It's not just portion sizes of food that up our intake of fat, sugar, and risky carbohydrates. Large portions of soda, fruit juice, and other beverages sweetened with high-fructose corn syrup or sugar add extra calories to our diets and extra fat to our bellies. Here's another Rescue, this time performed at Starbucks.

Risky! The 20-ounce (*venti*) White Chocolate Mocha with whole milk and whipped cream at Starbucks packs a staggering 620 calories—as much as a full-course meal.

Rescued! At 24 ounces, the Iced Skinny Flavored Latte made with fat-free milk contains 17 grams of carbohydrates and no fat. If you control carbs, opt for the 12-ounce size for 60 calories and 9 grams of carbs.

6. **Swap grease for greens.** To add fiber and healthy fats to your restaurant meal, skip the appetizers and order a salad with olive oil vinaigrette. (Request it "naked"—no cheese, bacon, or croutons.) As a side dish, opt for grilled or steamed veggies (with a drizzle of olive oil, if you like).

7. **Take the bread test.** If the bread is extraordinary—hot, crusty, whole grain—enjoy one slice, especially if it's sourdough. If it's the typical uninspired slightly warmed dinner rolls or Italian bread, take a pass. After all, you didn't go to a restaurant to eat bread and butter, did you? (If you're with people who want the bread, push the basket their way, so it's not in front of you.)

8. **Practice "safe servings."** If the restaurant you'll eat at is known for huge portions, split yours with a dining partner. Better yet, ask that it be wrapped to go before it's served to you.

9. **Watch for warning words.** Avoid like the plague any item described as crispy, crunchy, battered, fried, crusted, au gratin, scalloped, creamy, cheesy, large, grande, supreme, ultimate, sampler, combo, gringo, home style, or country style. Or

"granny's," for that matter. Perkins' Granny's Country Omelette, which comes with hash browns and three pancakes, hits you below the belt with 2,060 calories (a whole day's worth) and no less than 276 grams of carbs—equivalent to nearly a whole loaf of bread!

10. **Order like a pro.** You've got diabetes, like millions of other folks, and you're taking control by eating smart. So don't hesitate to ask your waitperson how menu items are prepared or request substitutions. If you're on a low-salt meal plan, ask that no salt be added to your food. Instead of ordering fries, request a double order of a vegetable. If you can't get a substitute, ask that the high-fat food be left off your plate. In short: speak up.

Rescue Your Fast-Food Meal

It's possible to eat healthfully at fast-food restaurants, even if you have diabetes. In this section, I highlight the Rescued options on each menu, rather than call out the Riskies, which tend to be similar (burgers as big as your head, items made with "crispy" chicken or fried fish, fries, fatty sauces and dressings, cheese, bacon, and so on).

The cheat sheet below sets you on the road to Rescue. As I said earlier, you can "order" your meal before you go. Some of these Web sites let you customize a meal (subtract cheese and dressings, for example), so you'll know exactly how many calories and how much fat and carbs your meal will contain before you hit the drive-thru window.

Arby's

Rescued! I can't call them "healthy," exactly. But healthier items on the sandwich menu include the regular Roast Beef sandwich (350 calories, 12 grams of fat, 39 grams of carbs) and the Melt sandwich (330 calories, 11 grams of fat, 40 grams of carbs). They're also healthier than any Market Fresh sandwich, all of which contain 330 to 380 calories and 64 to 71 grams of carbs from the bread alone. Add a chopped side salad (80 calories) with half a packet of balsamic vinaigrette dressing (65 calories) and you've got a filling meal for under 500 calories.

Burger King

Rescued! Opt for the TenderGrill Chicken Sandwich without mayo (360 calories and 7 grams of fat, 5 of them saturated) or, if available, the BK Veggie Burger without mayo (320 calories and 7 grams of fat, 1 of them saturated). Add a garden salad with the fat-free ranch dressing (150 calories) and you've Rescued this menu. If you really need a burger, the Whopper Jr. without mayo is a decent choice—260 calories and 10 grams of fat, 4 of them saturated.

Chick-fil-A

Rescued! This fast-food chain wisely features grilled offerings on its menu, shaving off a substantial amount of saturated fat and calories.

Go Fish—For Another Entrée

Seafood. The very word sounds healthy, doesn't it? I love seafood. How about you? If you do, you might be tempted to order the Seafood Sampler at Arthur Treacher's.

Throw this one back, folks. Here's how the entrée stacks up.

Calories: The sampler packs a staggering 3,378 calories—more than what you would get by eating three whole Pizza Hut Personal Panormous Pepperoni Pizzas all by yourself!

Carbs: Although seafood contains zero carbs, order this dish and you'll pack away 226 grams of carbohydrates. You'd have to cram down 15 slices of bread to get that many carbs!

Fat: The sampler contains 269 grams of fat, more than you'd consume in two full racks of Baby Back Ribs plus Aussie Fries at Outback.

Bottom line: This "seafood" platter wins my nomination for the "Diabetes Is Served" Restaurant Award.

The Chargrilled Chicken Sandwich is a healthy option at 290 calories, 4 grams of fat, 1 gram of saturated fat, and 3 grams of fiber. If it's a salad you crave, see the box below. The Chicken Salad Sandwich might sound healthy, but pass on it—the chunky bread and fat-filled mayo make it too high in calories (490), fat (19 grams), and carbs (55 grams) to Rescue it.

Fast-Food Salads: Risky and Rescued

If you're willing to order a salad at a fast-food place, I think you should be rewarded for your good intentions—by choosing a salad that's actually healthy. So I pulled together this list of Rescued and Risky fast-food salads. With the Riskies, I used the lowest-fat, lowest-calorie dressing available, as I suggest you do. Some of the Rescued salads become even healthier if you hold some of the optional extras.

Risky! These Riskies contain 10 to 17 grams of saturated fat, 36 to 56 grams of total fat, and up to 900 calories.

- **Wendy's BLT Cobb Salad** (with two packets of Light Classic Ranch dressing). Along with the salad greens and grape tomatoes, there's a fried chicken fillet, bacon, shredded Cheddar, and garlic croutons. It packs 760 calories, 55 grams of total fat, 17 grams of saturated fat, 4 grams of fiber, and 16 grams of carbs.

- **Arby's Crispy Chopped Farmhouse Salad** (with Balsamic Vinaigrette dressing). Even topped with the lightest dressing, because of the crispy popcorn chicken, bacon, and cheese, this salad packs 560 calories, 36 grams of total fat, 11 grams of saturated fat, and 31 grams of carbs.

- **Jack in the Box Chicken Club Salad** (with Bacon Ranch dressing). Same old unhealthy story: crispy chicken, croutons, bacon, cheese. This heart-stopper weighs in at 769 calories, 53 grams of total fat, 12 grams of saturated fat, and 38 grams of carbs.

KFC

Rescued! Stick with the grilled chicken and opt for green beans or a house salad with light dressing, and you've chosen a healthy meal that's low in fat and processed carbs. Other good options (although you'll want to nix them if you're on a low-sodium diet) include the Honey BBQ Sandwich (320 calories, 3.5 grams fat, 1 gram of saturated

---

Rescued! Rescued salads, from 130 to 280 calories as served, pack less than 10 grams of total fat and 4 grams or less of saturated fat.

- **Subway B.L.T. Salad.** For a restaurant with a reputation for healthy takeout, Subway offers surprisingly few Rescue-worthy salads. This variation on the classic bacon, lettuce, and tomato sandwich contains 130 calories, 8 grams of total fat, 3.5 grams of saturated fat, 3 grams of fiber, and only 7 grams of carbs.

- **Chick-fil-A Chargrilled Chicken Garden Salad** (with Reduced-Fat Berry Balsamic Vinaigrette). That fast-food restaurants offer grilled chicken items along with the Risky crispy variety does my heart good—and yours, too. This salad contains 250 calories, 8 grams of total fat, 4 grams of saturated fat, 4 grams of fiber, and 23 grams of carbs. *Mini-Rescue: Hold the croutons and you'll save calories, fat, and carbs.*

- **McDonald's Premium Southwest Salad with Grilled Chicken** (without dressing). Eating grilled chicken, not crispy, and holding the dressing make all the difference. This salad weighs in at 280 calories, 8.5 grams of total fat, 3 grams of saturated fat, 6 grams of fiber, and 20 grams of carbs. *Mini-Rescue: Hold the tortilla strips and you'll save calories, fat, and carbs.*

fat, and 3 grams of fiber); the KFC Snacker, ordered without sauce (260 calories, 9 grams of fat, 1.5 grams of saturated fat, and 2 grams of fiber); and the Roasted Caesar Salad, without croutons and with fat-free ranch dressing (250 calories, 8 grams of fat, 4.5 grams of saturated fat, 3 grams of fiber).

McDonald's

Rescued! If you hold the mayo, the Premium Grilled Chicken Classic Sandwich is a nutritious pick; it'll set you back 350 calories, 9 grams of fat, and 2 grams of saturated fat. Another good option: The Big 'N Tasty. *Men's Health*, the best restaurant detective in the business, calls it the best fast-food burger in America: "This generous patty edges out the iconic BK burger by a full 210 calories and brings a nice balance of protein, fat, and carbs to the table." Comes with lettuce, tomatoes, onion, and pickles. Or order the grilled-chicken salad (see "Fast-Food Salads: Risky and Rescued" on page 286).

Taco Bell

Rescued! Hold the cheese and sauces and order items "fresco style," a healthy, flavorful mix of tomatoes, onions, and cilantro. Good picks: The Fresco Chicken Soft Taco (150 calories, 3.5 grams of fat, 1 gram of saturated fat, and 2 grams of fiber) and Fresco Crunchy Taco (150 calories, 8 grams of fat, 2 grams of saturated fat, and 3 grams of fiber). This chain has a couple of healthy salads on its menu, too—just forgo the crispy salad "bowl" and order them fresco style.

Wendy's

Rescued! Try the Ultimate Chicken Grill—without the honey mustard sauce, it contains 330 calories, 4 grams of fat, 1 gram of saturated fat, and 1 gram of fiber. The small Chili (which I love) is also a good option—one serving packs just 210 calories and 6 grams of fiber but only 6 grams of fat (2.5 grams saturated). The beans in their chili are one of the healthiest foods you can eat, and they're not swimming in fatty dressing. Add a side salad with fat-free or vinaigrette dressing for less than 150 calories more.

Rescue Your Chain-Restaurant Meal

The order-before-you-go strategy is a good one when you plan to eat at a national chain, where the party atmosphere and big portions conspire to make you toss your good intentions out the window. Here's a big head start: examples of Risky and Rescued items at various chains.

Applebee's

Risky! I've already told you about one of their salads; the entrées aren't much healthier. Your goal is to sidestep the usual suspects—large portions, cheese, deep-fried items, high-fat sauces and dressing, and refined carbohydrates.

Rescued! Applebee's menu features several items created in partnership with Weight Watchers. What's more, the chain allows you to order half portions of some platters, which is great. A half portion of Grilled Chicken Caesar Salad, for instance, has just 410 calories instead of the 820 in the full order.

Applebee's also has a special menu section offering dishes with under 550 calories. You might want to try Sizzling Asian Shrimp & Broccoli (470 calories) or Grilled Dijon Chicken & Portobellos (also 470 calories). To see how much good you're doing yourself, consider that the same chain's Chicken Parmesan has 1,400 calories! You save nearly 1,000 calories and still get to enjoy a terrific chicken dish.

Chili's

Risky! *Bad* isn't a strong enough word for an "appetizer" at Chili's called Texas Cheese Fries with Chili and Ranch Dressing. It's packing 1,350 calories—nearly a full day's supply—and they call it an appetizer! But wait, that's a *half order*! The full order has 2,120 calories—as many as seven Egg McMuffins.

Another "appetizer" is called Hot Spinach and Artichoke Dip with Chips. Well, "spinach and artichokes" sounds healthy, as long as you don't realize that this has 1,610 calories—more than that half order of Texas Cheese Fries. Would you order an appetizer if you knew it had more calories than three Quarter Pounders with Cheese? Well, now you know!

Rescued! Skip the appetizers, watch portion sizes, and request that high-fat extras on salads—cheese, bacon bits, croutons, and the like—be held. I recommend either the beef or chicken fajitas, without tortillas and sides (390 and 360 calories, respectively). For sides, opt for two of these three: black beans (100 calories as served), avocado slices (full of healthy fat at only 80 calories as served), or fresh fruit (90 calories and 0 grams of saturated fat).

Cracker Barrel

Risky! Known for hearty country fare served in equally hearty portions, virtually all the offerings on its menu are served smothered in cheese, grease, or gravy. The sides aren't much help—mac and cheese, fried apples (?!), dumplings. And those buttermilk biscuits . . .

Rescued! Although Cracker Barrel is known for comfort food, you can still find healthy selections on the low-carb menu. Just pass up the items high in saturated fat, such as the bacon cheeseburger. And hold the cheese, please—it's also high in saturated fat. Might I suggest the grilled catfish (270 calories), turnip greens (98 calories), carrots (58 calories), and a slice of sourdough bread (110 calories)? At 536 calories, that meal is nutritional gold. Or opt for grilled roast beef (remove all visible fat), and pair it with a side of pinto beans and green beans or turnip greens (hold the butter).

Friendly's

Risky! The chain's BBQ Fronion Burger has 1,520 calories. Do a little searching and you'll discover that you could go to McDonald's and consume (if possible) a Quarter Pounder with Cheese, a large fries, an order of Chicken McNuggets, and a Hot Fudge Sundae—all for fewer calories.

The Apple Caramel Walnut Pancakes earned its high place by virtue of having an incredible 245 grams of carbohydrates. That's as much as you'd get if you could force—with the help of an evil machine—16 slices of bread down your gullet!

Rescued! Get the Half Turkey Club Supermelt (350 calories) and side garden salad (60 calories) with Lite Balsamic Vinaigrette

(180 calories). (Avoid the Bleu Cheese dressing, though. At 470 calories a serving, opting for it is like putting 10 strips of bacon on top of your salad!)

Olive Garden

Risky! At this chain, carb-heavy pasta isn't all there is to Italian cuisine. There are fat and huge portions, too. Unless you want to take in 1,320 calories, 80 grams of fat, and 30 grams of saturated fat, pass up the Grilled Sausage & Peppers Rustica—a family-style platter of Italian sausage with sautéed bell peppers over penne covered in mozzarella cheese and marinara sauce. Avoid the Tour of Italy pasta, too. You get lasagna, chicken parmigiana (breaded and fried), and fettuccine Alfredo, with a beef and Italian sausage meat sauce—for 1,450 calories, 97 grams of carbs, 74 grams of fat, and 33 grams of saturated fat.

Rescued! Look no further than the chain's Garden Fare menu, which has plenty of healthy options. Olive Garden even has lunch portions of pasta, all of which are under 500 calories. And some dishes contain even fewer than that—for example, the Venetian Apricot Chicken (290 calories; 4.5 grams of fat, 1.5 of them saturated; and 6 grams of fiber) and the Linguine alla Marinara (310 calories; 4 grams of fat, 1 of them saturated; and 5 grams of fiber). If you get one of the lower-calorie meals from this menu, pair it with a garden salad with light dressing or a cup of minestrone (100 calories).

Panera Bread

Risky! The reason you go to this chain—for the bread—is the same reason to proceed with extreme caution. Even a naked whole grain bagel contains 340 calories and 67 grams of carbs, and the healthy-sounding Mediterranean Veggie Sandwich on Tomato Basil bread packs 590 calories and 96 grams of carbs.

Rescued! I give this chain extra credit for offering half-size portions of many dishes, like a half Thai Chopped Chicken salad that has just 235 calories. Their Low-Fat Mango Smoothie sounds good, too, at just 230 calories.

Other Rescue candidates include half a Cuban Chicken Panini (430 calories), Cream of Chicken and Wild Rice Soup (310 calories), and Low-Fat Vegetarian Black Bean Soup (240 calories) paired with a Whole Grain Baguette side portion (180 calories).

Pizza Hut

Risky! Pizza is typically made with white flour and fatty meats and cheese, so you know what you're getting into. Then the portion sizes make things worse. Avoid the Personal Pan Pizzas, including the newer Panormous version, and the pasta selections. The heaviest hitter: the Meat Lover's pizza. One slice contains 330 calories—not bad—but 18 grams of fat, 7 of them saturated. Avoid the wings, too; the traditional ones are slightly less fatty and carb dense than the crispy bone-in wings, but that's not saying much.

Rescued! My picks include the Fit 'n Delicious 12-inch Green Pepper, Red Onion, and Diced Red Tomato Pizza (150 calories per slice) and Chicken, Mushroom, and Jalapeño Pizza (170 calories per slice). They're less calorie dense and contain less fat than the Thin 'N Crispy crust. If you stick to two slices, you'll do fine.

Red Lobster

Risky! Except for the jumbo shrimp cocktail, pass up most of the appetizers. For example, Crispy Calamari and Vegetables packs 1,520 calories and 97 grams of fat—nearly as much as four orders of large fries at Burger King. The word *crispy* is the warning. You wouldn't expect a seafood-and-vegetable platter to contain 115 grams of carbs (more than seven pieces of bread!), but this dish does, thanks to the crispy batter.

Rescued! Still, Red Lobster offers more healthy fare than most chains. An order of Peach-Bourbon BBQ Shrimp and Scallops contains just 490 calories, for instance. Or indulge safely with the Wood-Grilled Sirloin Surf and Turf—just 630 calories and a measly 21 grams of fat. In fact, the Ultimate Feast, under the Signature Combinations section of the menu, contains just 600 calories and 25 grams of carbs. Also, except for the carb-heavy Lobster and Shrimp Linguini Alfredo and the Maine Lobster and Shrimp Trio, the Menu Specials contain healthy fat, reasonable amounts of carbs, and fiber, if you order veggies on the side.

Ruby Tuesday

Risky! Overlook the appetizers, pasta classics, burgers, and sandwiches. And while it sounds healthy, pass up the Chicken and Broccoli Pasta, which weighs in at 1,521 calories, 92 grams of fat, and 96 grams of carbohydrates. It contains more calories than a couple of half racks of ribs!

Rescued! This chain has some nutritional gems hidden among the less-than-healthy fare. On the online nutritional information, they're called Smart Eating Choices. Here, among the plain grilled chicken or grilled sirloin (both under 290 calories each), you'll find New Orleans Seafood (365 calories) and White Bean Chicken Chili (300 calories). Add Fresh Steamed Broccoli (53 calories). The Petite Lunch Plates are also good options. For example, the grilled chicken salad, shrimp scampi, and creole catch are all under 380 calories. Stick with Balsamic Vinaigrette Dressing (40 calories per serving), or use less dressing and add salsa (8 calories per serving) for a flavorful treat.

Oatmeal . . . or Elvis?

If you're tempted to drink your lunch on a hot day, Planet Smoothie is a good chain to visit. But first, answer this question: Which of the following smoothies has the most calories?

   a) Chocolate Elvis
   b) Screamsicle
   c) Oatmeal
   d) Chocolate Chimp Workout Blast

You could see this coming: Oatmeal has the most, at 490 calories (nearly as much as Chocolate Chimp and Screamsicle put together). So if you're not embarrassed to order a Chocolate Chimp Workout Blast, that's a fine choice.

Rescue Ethnic Cuisine, Too

Ethnic cuisine, especially Asian cuisine, has a reputation for being healthy. But it's still possible to get ambushed. Exhibit A: P.F. Chang's.

The Almond & Cashew Chicken Lunch Bowl with brown rice (535 calories) sounds great on first reading of the chain's nutrition information. Look again. This is actually a half portion of what they serve. Checking their menu, there's not a word about this being a two-portion serving. So what you'll get actually packs more than 1,070 calories—more than you'd get in a huge 1-pound sirloin steak, plus a small fries!

Because ethnic cuisine isn't prepared the same way at every restaurant, the lists below can't be as specific as those for fast-food places and national chains. Still, more and more ethnic restaurants have placed their menus online, with descriptions of the items. So if you can, log on and order before you go.

Chinese

Risky! Egg rolls, spare ribs, fried dumplings, pork lo mein, fried rice, moo shu, General Tso's chicken, sweet-and-sour pork, wonton soup

Rescued! Steamed or stir-fried seafood, chicken, bean curd, or vegetable dishes—plus steamed brown rice, if it's available. Request that your dish be prepared with less oil; if you're watching your salt intake, request that the cook leave out soy sauce and MSG. At 600 calories, moo goo gai pan is a good choice, as is shrimp with lobster sauce (400 calories). The guys at *Men's Health* vote for Peking duck, because most of the fat has been rendered out to make the skin extra crispy.

Smart choice: A spring roll has half the calories of an egg roll (100 versus 200). Also, marinades and sauces often contain high levels of sodium and sugar, so request that the chef use less—and hold the cornstarch, too.

Greek and Middle Eastern

Risky! Moussaka (lamb and beef casserole) and other creamy or cheesy entrées, gyros, falafel, baklava (Greek pastry)

Rescued! Greek salad; roast lamb shish kebab (all visible fat removed); minty, spicy tabbouleh (bulgur wheat) with grilled chicken; *plaki* (fish cooked in tomatoes and onions; hold the cheese); *tzatziki* (yogurt and cucumber sauce); baba ghannouj, a delicious puree of eggplant flavored with tahini, lemon juice, and fresh herbs

Smart choice: To add heart-healthy veggies and fiber to your meal, choose appetizers made with chickpeas, like hummus, as well as eggplant, tomatoes, and grains, such as tabbouleh.

Indian

Risky! Dishes prepared with high-fat ingredients like clarified butter (called ghee) and coconut milk (fortunately, menus often specify), *poori* (fried, puffy bread)

Rescued! Tandoori—meats, poultry, or fish cooked in a clay oven with spices and no added fats—and vegetable curries, if they're not prepared with ghee

Smart choice: Shrimp or fish tandoori with the flavorful yogurt-based sauce called *raita*

Italian

Risky! Garlic bread/breadsticks, pasta sauces made with meat (Bolognese) or cheese (Alfredo), fried calamari, pastas stuffed with cheese, veal/chicken or eggplant Parmesan

Rescued! Light sauces like marinara, primavera, clam, or marsala (wine, mushrooms, beef stock); *branzino*; sea bass; mussels *fra diavolo*

Smart choice: Ask your waitperson if you can order pasta in a smaller (lunch) portion, regardless of the time of day. If you must have bread, limit yourself to one slice, dipped in olive oil rather than spread with butter.

Japanese

Risky! Any kind of tempura, fried *gyoza* (the Japanese version of Chinese pot stickers) or fried wonton, *agedashi* tofu (deep-fried tofu), *niku-itame* (stir-fried pork), specialty rolls (may have more ingredients than basic rolls)

Rescued! Seaweed salad, miso soup, broiled sea bass (or any broiled fish), yakitori (grilled chicken), steamed gyoza, sushi, *nigiri*, sashimi, edamame, *oshitoshi* (steamed spinach)

Smart choice: Like sushi? See the box above. If you can't get sushi with brown rice, opt for a tuna roll (184 calories and 2 grams of fat) or an avocado roll—at just 140 calories, it has a big 6 grams of fiber.

Mexican

Risky! Chips, fried tacos, refried beans, quesadillas, chimichangas, enchiladas, beef burritos

Rescued! Black beans, black bean soup, grilled shrimp, grilled chicken or fish. Another delicious option: chicken or shrimp fajitas—marinated chicken or shrimp grilled with onions and green peppers and served with lettuce and diced tomatoes. Opt for one whole grain corn or whole wheat tortilla instead of one made with white flour, and swap the sour cream and guacamole for flavorful salsa.

Smart choice: Tell your waitperson not to bring fried tortilla chips to your table. They go down easy, but they're just as unhealthy as white bread!

Thai

Risky! Heavy sauces and deep-fried items, including fried spring rolls, dishes with coconut milk, peanuts, cashews and peanut sauce, duck, or *tom ka gai* (coconut chicken soup)

Rescued! Steamed spring rolls, hot-and-sour soup, vegetable stir-fries (ask that they be prepared with very little vegetable oil rather than coconut oil or lard)

Smart choice: Start with a papaya salad—crisp, pleasantly sweet/tart shredded fruit, chile-lime dressing on the side—followed by a *satay* (grilled skewer of meat or poultry). Satays come with dipping sauces; use them sparingly.

Part 3

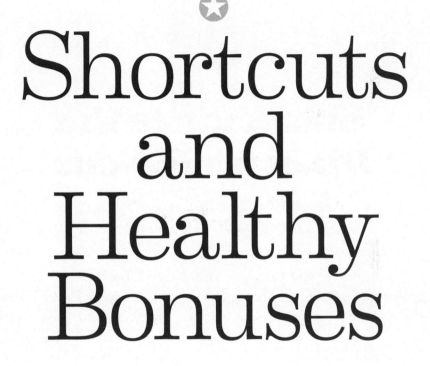

Shortcuts and Healthy Bonuses

Shortcuts to the Diabetes Rescue

Simple Moves to Turbocharge Your Health Protection

Besides the diet guidance you've already read, there are a number of simple steps you can take that may do a world of good for your diabetes defense strategy. All of these have been proven scientifically to help prevent or control diabetes. Of course, these are in addition to your doctor's advice about blood sugar control, medications, and more. You may be surprised to see how easy some of these tips are—and the tremendous extent to which they can help add to your health protection!

Aspirin: Medicine Cabinet Diabetes Protection

You don't often hear *aspirin* and *diabetes* in the same sentence. But now you have, and you could use the information that follows to literally save your life.

The key is that the number one health threat facing a person with

300

diabetes is an "event" affecting the heart and circulatory system. The risk is twice as high as that facing a person the same age without diabetes. Low-dose aspirin is very good at blocking these life-threatening events.

In one study, more than 6,000 people who were deemed at high risk of coronary disease were followed for 3 years. Those who'd taken daily aspirin were 44 percent less likely to die of any cause.

What about people who have diabetes—do they respond the same way? One group that tackled this question was composed of doctors at a Department of Veteran Affairs health center. They found that 66 percent of their patients with diabetes were taking aspirin. Compared with patients who had not taken aspirin, these folks were far less likely to have heart problems.

In fact, the doctors reported this: "We estimate for this population that increasing daily aspirin use to 90 percent [versus 66 percent] could prevent an additional 11,000 heart attacks and potentially save more than 8,000 lives."

The 2010 Fremantle Diabetes Study confirmed the huge upside of low-dose aspirin for people with diabetes. Following more than 651 people for 10 years, the researchers found that those who'd been taking aspirin when the project began were 47 percent less likely to have died from any cause at all and 70 percent less likely to die from cardiovascular disease.

Does it seem amazing to you that an inexpensive over-the-counter drug like aspirin can have such a profound protective effect? And that you haven't heard more about it? It does to me!

One more thing: You should check with your physician before beginning low-dose aspirin. It's not for everybody. If you have a history of gastrointestinal bleeding or are taking certain other drugs—especially those that thin the blood to prevent dangerous clotting, like warfarin—you may be told to skip aspirin. But please, do ask!

Breakfast: The Antidiabetes Meal

Just for the heck of it, I searched for "tips to prevent diabetes" and visited numerous health-related Internet sites to see if they mention the topic of this Shortcut to the Diabetes Rescue. None did—which makes eating breakfast one of the many health "secrets" you're learning about in this book!

Fact: People who eat breakfast regularly are 30 to 50 percent less likely to be obese or develop diabetes than folks who usually skip it.

A study of thousands of young adults found that breakfast skippers were much more likely to be obese and have insulin resistance syndrome. People with that problem may not have diabetes, but their bodies cannot handle glucose efficiently, and they are at higher risk of both diabetes and heart disease.

The link between eating breakfast and not being overweight or obese is especially strong. And since excess pounds are a major risk for diabetes, breakfast seems like more than just another meal.

And the best breakfast is . . . A researcher from Michigan State University found that women who regularly ate breakfast were 24 percent less likely to be overweight than women who skipped it. And if they ate cereal as part of breakfast, their risk was even lower—30 percent less.

That's women. What about men? It works for them, too. In another study, following more than 20,000 men for 10 years, scientists found that breakfast eaters were much less likely to gain 11 pounds over a 10-year period. Compared with breakfast skippers, their reduced risk was 23 percent—almost identical to the protection that women receive.

I've made my point, but I'm going to mention one other study because it reveals at least two fascinating facts about breakfast. A study called EAT (Eating Among Teens) followed thousands of adolescents for 5 years, keeping track of their dietary habits and weight. The finding—no surprise—was that there was a direct "dose response" relationship between eating breakfast and weight gain adjusted for height. The more often kids ate breakfast, the less likely they were to become fat.

But the researchers also found that teens who were trying to lose weight were the ones most likely to skip breakfast—in hopes of losing weight! Sadly, that only made them fatter. (You have to wonder how many adults fall into the same trap.)

There was another important finding—or, rather, lack of finding. The researchers analyzed a bunch of dietary factors that might explain the healthful effect of eating breakfast and confessed they couldn't pin down any special reasons. There seems to be something about the antifatness power of eating breakfast that goes beyond the sheer nutrients consumed. So if anyone asks you why you always eat breakfast to protect against weight gain and diabetes, you can say, "It's a bit of a mystery, actually!"

No mystery about what types of cereal to choose, though. Whole grain cold cereals and hot cereals like oatmeal (especially Irish oatmeal) are among the best. Steer clear of cornflakes, puffed cereals, and Chex cereal, as they all tend to spike blood sugar.

Chocolate: Melt-in-Your-Mouth "Medicine"

Chocolate isn't part of the traditional Mediterranean Diet. But the fact is, a little bit can go a long way toward saving your life—so it's part of the Diabetes Rescue Diet!

Prompted by increasing evidence that chocolate is good for the heart, health researchers studied the diets and presence of coronary heart disease in 4,970 people ages 25 to 93. What the researchers discovered: Compared with people who never ate chocolate, those who had some one to four times a week had 26 percent less heart disease. Those who ate chocolate more than five times a week had 57 percent less incidence of heart disease.

And know this: It turned out that people who ate nonchocolate candy five or more times week not only didn't benefit, they suffered, with 49 percent more cases of heart disease.

Perhaps you think this is just crazy. Cutting your risk of heart disease more than half . . . with chocolate? Perhaps people who love chocolate are somehow healthier, younger, or otherwise protected. The researchers thought the same thing and therefore adjusted their numbers to account for the effects of age, sex, family history of heart disease, smoking, exercise, and all sorts of other factors. The results they reported take all that into consideration, strongly suggesting that it was chocolate and not something else that produced the tremendous health effect.

Perhaps you suspect this study was sponsored by the company in Hershey, Pennsylvania, and is therefore biased. That's not the case: The research was actually part of the National Heart, Lung, and Blood Institute (NHLBI) Family Heart Study and carried out by scientists from Harvard Medical School and two other medical centers.

Chocolate—especially dark chocolate—is known to have natural compounds that promote health. But the finding that it can reduce risk of heart disease by more than half seems extraordinary. For people with diabetes, who are at higher risk, it seems like a breakthrough finding that should be trumpeted from the rooftops. But the only trumpeting you're likely to hear is right here. The study was published in a leading journal in 2011 and followed by silence from the government that sponsored it.

I'm not much for conspiracy theories, but my guess is that health experts in general are following the philosophy of "You want the truth? You can't *handle* the truth!" In other words, publicizing this news would encourage people to abandon fruits and vegetables and stuff themselves with chocolate candies.

I have more faith in you than that. It seems that small portions of dark chocolate can promote and protect health, so if you'd like some, just keep the portion modest. Keep reading and you'll see how little you may need.

If you haven't heard about chocolate and hypertension, here's another study to consider: In 2010, an Australian team analyzed 15 different studies done on the relation between flavonols (the ingredients in chocolate believed to help blood vessels dilate) and blood pressure and found that, yes, it works. They reported that after evaluating all the different studies, it could be said that nibbling chocolate tends to lower systolic blood pressure about 5 points—about the same as 30 minutes of physical activity a day.

My suggestion: How about walking *and* having a little bit of chocolate?

There may be more than blood pressure involved here. In 2010, the journal *Diabetic Medicine* published a study examining the effect of chocolate on cholesterol and other risk factors in patients with type 2 diabetes. The finding: After 8 weeks on a diet including about 1½ ounces of polyphenol-rich (dark) chocolate a day, patients had a notable increase in HDL ("good") cholesterol, indicating less risk of clogged arteries. And there was no change in weight, insulin resistance, or glucose control.

If your doctor has told you that your HDL levels are on the low side, you might want to ask about this. In any event, remember that added calories from chocolate should be subtracted from other foods.

What if you've had a heart attack already? Could chocolate benefit your health? You'll want to consult with your cardiologist on that, but meanwhile, consider this mind-blowing fact: In Stockholm, Sweden, doctors examined the diets of people who had had a heart attack and followed their health outcomes for 8 years. One of the questions the doctors asked was about chocolate consumption.

The somewhat amazing finding was that the more chocolate the patients ate, the less likely they were to die from another heart problem. Compared with people who never ate chocolate, those who did so less than once a month were 27 percent less likely to die from cardiac causes. Those who ate chocolate up to once a week were 44 percent

---

Chocolate Saves Seniors!

Should you give Uncle John some chocolates for his birthday? Read this and decide.

In the Netherlands, 470 "elderly" (I hate that word!) men were followed as part of the Zutphen Elderly Study. Over a period of 15 years, their diets were checked repeatedly and their health ascertained.

When the men were divided into three groups based on the amount of cocoa they ate (low, medium, high) from all sources, those in the top group were 50 percent less likely to die from heart problems and 47 percent less likely to die from any cause at all.

The idea that chocolate can cut the risk of death in half for seniors sounds crazy. But it fits in perfectly with other research, and now that you've read all about chocolate and health, it doesn't seem that crazy, does it?

---

less likely to die. And those who indulged twice a week or more were 66 percent less likely to die! Consumption of any other kind of candy had no effect at all on risk.

Interestingly, patients with diabetes were excluded from the study, because, it was figured, they'd probably been counseled to avoid all sweets, including chocolate.

Coffee: Go to "Joe" to Defeat Diabetes

You could read all the diabetes brochures in your doctor's office, go to lectures about diabetes at the community center, or scan a dozen Internet articles about preventing diabetes, and I'd bet you wouldn't find one word about the health-saving effect of coffee.

Coffee? Good for you? Yes. And get this: Coffee may be better at preventing diabetes than one of the most widely used and respected prescription drugs.

One study, done in the Netherlands in 2009, found that people who drank three or more cups of coffee a day reduced their risk of diabetes by a mighty 42 percent.

In 2005, the *Journal of the American Medical Association* published a study that involved more than 193,000 people. The finding: People who drank four to six cups of coffee a day were one-third less likely to develop diabetes, compared with those who drank zero to two cups a day. The authors added that the trend of more coffee, less diabetes held up in the United States, northern Europe, southern Europe, and Japan as well.

Still another study pegged the reduced rate of diabetes with drinking four cups of joe a day at 47 percent—nearly half!

But here's the study that interests me most, because it suggests that coffee may have powers comparable or even superior to a prescription drug. Researchers from the Department of Family and Preventive Medicine at the University of California, San Diego, enrolled 910 people without diabetes in a study that went on for 8 years. But they added something special: Each participant was given a standard test to see if they had what's called impaired glucose tolerance. People with this problem are much more likely to develop type 2 diabetes than the average person.

At the end of the 8 years, the doctors found that past drinkers of coffee had 64 percent less risk of developing diabetes; current coffee drinkers, 62 percent less risk. Among people who'd been ID'd as having trouble with sugar metabolism, coffee drinkers also reduced the risk of diabetes by 62 to 64 percent!

That reminded me of the famous Diabetes Prevention Project, done in the 1990s. It, too, dealt with people who had impaired glucose tolerance. But this study involved the drug metformin (brand name: Glucophage—which means "sugar eater") instead of coffee.

Patients who didn't get the drug were put on either an intensive lifestyle-change program or dummy pills (placebos). After several years, the project was halted prematurely—because both treatments were working so well, it seemed inhumane to let anyone take dummy pills!

How effective was metformin? It reduced cases of diagnosed diabetes by a hefty 31 percent. Today, this Rx drug is very widely prescribed and highly respected. But consider this: People in the San Diego study with the same impaired glucose tolerance reduced their chances of developing diabetes by 62 to 64 percent—twice the protection of the drug—with . . . coffee!

Now, I'm not advocating that you start drinking three or four cups of coffee a day. For one thing, all these studies involved people who'd been drinking coffee for years, and short-term effects could be different. The caffeine could bother you. (Some studies show that coffee has to contain caffeine to fight diabetes; other studies, oddly, show decaf doing a comparable job.) Or maybe you're a tea lover. (Tea may help like coffee, some studies suggest; others disagree.)

What I'm saying is that if you drink a few cups of coffee, you shouldn't worry that it's doing you harm, unless your doctor tells you otherwise. If you do like coffee and the caffeine isn't a problem, you might try adding a cup or so a day. At around 4:00 p.m., my wife and I often prepare homemade lattes with strong French roast coffee and 1 percent milk. Although, to be honest, it's more for our minds than our health!

What if you have diabetes? Is coffee still good or at least okay?

Researchers from the United States, Spain, and China looked into this question, targeting men with type 2 diabetes, and published their findings in 2009. They found that men with diabetes who drank four or more cups of coffee a day had a 20 percent lower risk of death from all causes than nondrinkers, as well as a 12 percent lower risk of cardiovascular disease. Caffeine intake made no difference one way or the other, suggesting that decaf might be a helper, too.

Driving with Diabetes: Two Ways to Stay Safer

Whether you're on insulin, oral drugs, or both, there is always the risk of hypoglycemia (too-low blood sugar). The worst time to go "hypo" is when you're driving—and it happens, especially to people with type 1 diabetes, who are completely dependent on insulin to control their blood sugar.

An international study group visited diabetes specialty clinics in seven US and four European cities and had patients (and their spouses) fill out anonymous questionnaires about their driving experiences. The finding: During the previous 2 years, people with type 1 diabetes had "significantly more crashes and moving violations; episodes of hypoglycemic stupor, requiring assistance; and mild hypoglycemia" than type 2 drivers—or nondiabetic spouses. Scary statistic: Nineteen percent of type 1 drivers reported having at least one crash over the previous 2 years!

Can anything be done to reduce this danger? Yes—big time! The authors of the study point to a blood glucose awareness program that teaches you to anticipate, prevent, detect, and treat hypoglycemia. It's been shown to reduce crashes and moving violations by two-thirds at longtime follow-up.

If you can't enroll in such a program, here are two simple guidelines urged for people with type 1 diabetes.

1. Take your blood sugar, and if it's under 90 milligrams, don't drive. Tests show that your ability to drive becomes impaired at about 65 milligrams, so this leaves you a safety margin.

2. If you feel you're going too low while driving, pull over to a safe

spot immediately, consume some fast-acting carbohydrates, and don't resume driving until your blood sugar and mental state return to normal. Your best bet for those fast-acting carbs is glucose tablets, which you can keep in the storage bin next to the driver's seat. (See "Low Blood Sugar: Bounce Back in Less Than 15 Minutes" on page 312 for information.)

I don't think you should feel immune to the danger of low blood sugar behind the wheel if you have type 2 diabetes, rather than type 1, especially if insulin is part of your regimen. A study done in Scotland found that hypoglycemia requiring emergency assistance from health personnel was as common among people with type 2 diabetes who took insulin as among those with type 1.

Eggs: Have Diabetes?
Be Eggs-tra Careful!

Eggs used to be condemned as heart-stoppers because of their cholesterol and saturated fat. They're pretty much off the hook now, since research has found no association between heart disease and eating eggs. But for you—a person trying to avoid diabetes or already coping with it—the story could be different.

Research done at Harvard Medical School and other health centers found that eating eggs on a regular basis seems to increase the risk of developing diabetes. Eggs on Sunday morning doesn't seem like a serious risk, but in the study, men who ate an egg or more every day were found to have a 58 percent increased risk of being diagnosed.

Do eggs raise blood sugar? Some research says yes, some says no. At this point, the reason for the connection between eggs and diabetes is simply unknown. The doctors who wrote the report in *Diabetes Care* suggest that the smart thing to do is make eggs a not-every-day food.

What if you are currently dealing with diabetes? The same advice to go easy on eggs could be right for you, too—maybe even more so. Other research has revealed that men who eat as few as two eggs a week have double the chance of developing heart disease as men who eat less than one egg a week. For women, the increased risk was about half as much but still a little scary.

The interesting—*annoying*—thing is that this connection was found only in folks with type 2 diabetes! I used to eat egg salad sandwiches for lunch a few times a week. I gave it up after seeing this research and now favor tuna salad and tomato on whole wheat. I don't like eggs *that* much!

Fasting: Not So Fast!

Many people with diabetes are faced with a dilemma during holy days that involve fasting. Jewish people have several holy days, like Yom Kippur, during which they are not to eat—or drink—anything for 24 hours. Ramadan, the Muslim holy period, calls for fasting and not drinking from sunup to sundown for a whole month. Many people with diabetes observe these fasts—whether it's safe for them to do so or not—so my purpose here is to help you make sure your holy day doesn't wind up with you in a hospital.

Is the threat really that serious? Well, it's not trivial when you look at medical records.

An international group of physicians of the Muslim faith reported in the medical journal *Diabetes Care* that people with type 1 diabetes who fast during Ramadan have nearly five times the risk of being hospitalized because of severe hypoglycemia (low blood sugar) as those with type 1 who don't fast.

People who have the more common type 2 diabetes have a $7\frac{1}{2}$ times higher risk of winding up in the hospital. The physicians suggest that the real risk is even greater. Reason: These statistics from a very large study don't include people who became hypoglycemic but were helped to recover through the timely actions of a friend, rather than medical personnel.

You could see that coming. Even without fasting, many people with diabetes experience occasional bouts of serious low blood sugar. But oddly, fasting can also lead to serious high blood sugar.

According to the same large study, people with diabetes who observe the Ramadan fast are five times more likely to be hospitalized because of hyperglycemia (high blood sugar). The doctors suggest two possible reasons for this: One is cutting back excessively on medications that control sugars. The other is "the common practice of ingesting large amounts of food rich in carbohydrates and fat, especially at the sunset meal" (when eating is allowed again). They advise that a fast be broken immediately if blood sugar drops lower than 60 milligrams or goes higher than 300 milligrams.

But here's the most important thing of all: Both the Bible and the Koran make it clear that if you have a health problem that makes fasting and not drinking dangerous, you're officially excused. And if you have diabetes, that means you!

If you're still determined to fast, the doctors suggest speaking to your physician, who is familiar with your history. And they advise their fellow physicians to caution any person whose sugars are poorly controlled or who can't take blood sugar tests "multiple times" during the day not to fast.

Flu Shots: Go Shopping, Save Your Life

If you have diabetes, you should know that an annual vaccine is important. Here's proof: A study in England during two flu epidemics found that people with diabetes who'd gotten their vaccinations were 79 percent less likely to wind up in a hospital.

That flu shot can even help prevent a heart attack! Since people with diabetes are at a heightened risk of heart trouble, it makes sense to take advantage of any simple way to gain protection. A study of adults age 40 and over who got flu vaccine shots found they were 19 percent less likely to have a first heart attack in the next year.

And get that shot early. Those who were vaccinated from September to mid-November lowered their risk even more—by 21 percent.

I've gotten shots at my gym, my doctor's office, and a community center, but this year was the easiest of all. My wife and I went into a Sam's Club to stock up on staples and discovered they were giving flu shots!

Low Blood Sugar: Bounce Back in Less Than 15 Minutes

People who take oral meds or insulin (or both) have to be aware of the danger of hypoglycemia—low blood sugar. You may have heard about using candy, juice, soda, or sugar pills to get your sugar up out of the danger zone. But which is best?

French doctors decided to compare the effects of glucose and sucrose in various forms—including tablets, gels, or drinks—and orange juice. Volunteers with diabetes who had recently taken their insulin were shot up with more insulin to induce hypoglycemia. When they began to experience symptoms or asked for treatment, they were give one of the "antidotes" as 15 grams of carbohydrates.

In the winner's circle were glucose and sucrose in tablet or drink form. The gels didn't perform well. And the OJ washed out: Ten minutes after consumption of the sugars, blood sugar came up nicely, but with OJ, almost nothing happened. By the 14-minute mark, the sugar pills had resolved all symptoms of hypoglycemia.

The authors suggest that glucose tablets are more palatable than sucrose, so you may want to go that way. Note that each pill may have only 4 grams of carbs, so think four tablets.

Personal suggestion: Get them out of the big awkward bottle and put them into little plastic bags you keep in your car, jacket pocket, walking-around belt pack, and bedroom.

Massage: More Than a Feel-Good Experience?

If you feel you need an excuse to plunk down some money for a massage, I've got a good one for you: It could help lower your blood sugar.

A study at a first-rate medical facility—the Center of Family Medicine in Stockholm, Sweden—ran a small pilot study to see if women with diabetes who were given a series of massage sessions would show any benefit. The group was small (just 11 women), and they received 60-minute full-body massages once a week for 10 weeks. The massages were gentle—no kneading or manipulating muscle under the skin. Many different tests and measurements were taken before the project got under way, after each session, and at the end of the trial.

After 10 weeks, the women's A1c levels went down, on average, from 6.3 percent to 5.4 percent—which is a very large drop. Interestingly, three women were taken off the trial because their blood sugar was going too low, and their own doctors had to change their medications. What's most impressive is that 12 weeks after the massages ended, the A1c levels were holding steady at the new lower range.

The researchers noted that there were no major changes in physical activity and no drop in insulin resistance to explain the improvements. There was a small reduction in levels of the stress hormone cortisol, but that didn't appear to fully explain the change. It seems there is something special about massage, though the researchers couldn't pinpoint exactly what it is.

Now, this was a small pilot study, conducted back in 2004, so you can't count on the results as being "proven." There hasn't been a larger follow-up study, which means the pilot study remains just a "suggestion," not proof of a reliable treatment.

On the other hand, the clinic that did the research is part of the world-renowned Karolinska Institute, which handles the awarding of the Nobel Prize in Physiology or Medicine. So it's not exactly a massage parlor! And really, can you imagine any side effects other than complete relaxation and loose muscles?

Moisturizer: Save Your Feet in 60 Seconds

If you have diabetes, you should be well aware that your feet need special care. Here's a simple tip that can help prevent a disaster: Dry skin (doctors call it xerosis) is very common among people with diabetes, especially around their heels. One study found that 82 percent of a group of people with diabetes had dryness, cracks, and fissures on their feet.

This is not good. Those cracks can lead to ulcerations, which can then become infected. If blood sugar is high, it can feed the bacteria, and the result can be amputation.

There are a number of things you should do to protect your feet, but here's one simple way to help stop the progression to amputation: Use moisturizer! Apply it every day after bathing. An especially effective and cheap choice is simple petroleum jelly. Or use a less messy one. A dermatologist once recommended Curel to me, so that's what I use.

But now listen up: When you apply moisturizer, you might be tempted to rub some in between your toes. Don't! It isn't absorbed well, and the skin can become too soft, which can lead to damage. In fact, you should be extra careful to dry between your toes after bathing.

Neuropathy of the Feet:
Walk Away from It—In Less Than
an Hour a Day

A very common complication of diabetes is diabetic peripheral neuropathy (DPN), which can be very troublesome. There are two kinds of DPN: With sensory neuropathy, your feet lose sensation, which is dangerous because you may not be aware of things causing injury to your feet. With motor neuropathy, your footing becomes unsure. You may have trouble standing or walking. Because of their stumbling, people with this problem face 15 times the normal risk of being injured when they walk. Some people have both forms of DPN, making matters worse.

There is no definitive treatment for DPN, but a recent trial found that you can stop this problem in its tracks—before it stops *you* in your tracks! Researchers divided 78 patients, none of whom had DPN, into two groups. One group did nothing special, while the other group participated in a supervised walking program and logged a total of 4 hours of brisk treadmill walking each week. After 4 years, there was a striking difference between the two groups. Among the nonwalkers, the incidence of motor neuropathy was 17 percent; in the walkers, *zero percent*. For sensory neuropathy, the nonwalkers had 29.8 percent incidence; the walkers, just 6.45 percent.

The Diabetes Rescue Diet recommends nearly this much walking, but to hit 4 hours a week, you might need to add a bit more each day.

An average of 40 minutes a day will take you to the 4-hour program that worked so well.

Another way to prevent or reduce DPN problems is by taking strict control of your blood sugar. If you currently have DPN, you should certainly talk with your doctor before launching a walking program.

Pizza: Three Steps to the Perfect Pie?

There's something about pizza that is not friendly to blood sugar control. Many people with diabetes who test their sugars regularly have noticed this—and complained bitterly. "Never touch the stuff—it causes my blood sugar to go crazy!" is a typical comment from those susceptible to the pizza problem. I'm going to suggest a possible way to rescue yourself from the tragedy of a no-pizza lifestyle or worrying whenever you enjoy it. But first let's look at some pizza science.

Back in 1993, researchers at Yale–New Haven Hospital in Connecticut fed either pizza or a high-glycemic meal (foods known to create fast or high increases in blood sugar, such as cake, white bread, and baked potatoes) to a group of men with well-controlled type 1 diabetes.

The researchers already knew that eating pizza was associated with high postmeal sugar rises, but wanted to discover if this was due to simply overeating or something peculiar about pizza. They made sure the meals had the same amount of carbohydrates, fat, and protein, so you wouldn't expect that much difference in glucose response.

After the first few hours, both meals caused blood sugar to rise equally. But then the pizza meal caused levels to keep rising, hour after hour—like an evil Energizer bunny—with the effect continuing for 4 to 9 hours after eating.

Here's an approach I think should reduce the problem of pizza, even though there is no specific research proving it. First, go for a thin crust. Domino's thin-crust pizza has just half the carbs as hand tossed (67 grams versus 139) in a small pie. The suggested thin-crust serving is one-quarter of a pie, so the total carbs are less than 18 grams—a tad more than in one slice of bread. Since carbs are the primary force behind rising sugar, that move should help a lot.

For the cheese topping, go for feta, which adds just 60 calories to a whole pie and has very little fat—only 4 grams. (Italian sausage topping has 21 grams!) Then add a few vegetable toppings like bell peppers, onions, garlic, or mushrooms. Maybe, just maybe, in the context of diabetes, you have the perfect pizza!

Shoes: Ask This Question, Save Your Feet

The next time you visit your podiatrist, instead of immediately taking off your shoes, leave them on and ask her or him if they fit properly. You may think they do, but you could be wrong—really wrong!

When podiatrists at a Veteran's Affairs clinic examined hundreds of patients, including many with diabetes, they found that only one in four wore appropriate-size shoes. But those who had diabetic foot ulcers were five times more likely to be wearing poorly fitting shoes than other patients who also had diabetes but no wounds.

In Dundee, Scotland, doctors at a diabetes clinic checked the footwear of patients and found almost exactly the same thing: Only 20 percent of patients had shoes that fit correctly, both sitting and standing. The doctors pointed out that improper fit was not due to sensory neuropathy—the loss of sensation in the feet—or any other special factor. Bad judgment seemed the reason. Their conclusion: "Many patients with diabetes wear shoes that do not fit, particularly *shoes that are too narrow for their foot width*." (Emphasis added.)

Given the seriousness of foot ulcers, get your shoes checked out!

Sleep Deficiency: The "5 Minute" Remedy That Reduces Diabetes Risk

The idea that improving your sleep habits could make a major difference in your risk of developing diabetes sounds, well, strange. The truth is that millions of people could bolster their defense against this widespread disease by simply deciding to go to bed earlier.

In a 2009 medical study, people who slept just 7 or fewer hours a night were more than twice as likely to develop diabetes as people who slept at least 8 hours. More than doubling your risk is serious stuff—women who smoke a pack a day, for instance, have less than half that degree of increased risk of diabetes.

Now, you might suspect that some hidden factors were at risk here. Maybe short sleepers had other problems that encouraged diabetes, such as impaired glucose control or being heavier. But even after accounting for those and other factors, the conclusion was that short-changing yourself on sleep is "an independent risk factor" for diabetes.

And it's easy to be burdened by that risk, because, as one scientist points out, "over the past 40 years, sleep duration has decreased by almost 2 hours." But what exactly is the connection between a little less sleep and a much greater risk of diabetes? The answer is that a deficiency of sleep literally changes your body chemistry in ways that push you toward diabetes.

One study had a group of healthy young people shorten their sleep from 8 to 6 hours a night. After a week, researchers noted an upsurge in production of proinflammatory cytokines—compounds known to encourage diabetes and its complications to the extent that one scientist says flatly, "Diabetes and inflammation are inseparable."

More research on sleep deficiency found that it reduces production of a hormone that helps control appetite and increases another that promotes appetite—especially for junk food!

It's not surprising that a very large study found a definite relationship between getting less than 7 hours of sleep and being obese: The less sleep, the higher the body mass. And, of course, since obesity is a major contributor to diabetes risk, that seems to cement the sleep deficiency–diabetes link. I took special interest in the fact that the link remained strong even after people with insomnia were excluded. This means that simply choosing to sleep less than the optimal amount is the main problem, not tossing and turning all night. The researchers' conclusion is worth quoting: "Voluntary sleep restriction may contribute to the large public health burden of DM [diabetes mellitus]."

If it's voluntary, that means you can change it, without necessarily seeking help or sleeping pills. Here's one suggestion: Go to bed about 5 minutes earlier every night for a few weeks. Simple, but it worked for me!

Smoking: Quitting—The Fast Track to Decreasing Risk

You already know that smoking increases your risk of heart disease and cancer. But diabetes?

Researchers at the Harvard School of Public Health asked themselves that same question and came up with a surprising answer. After following a group of nurses over the years, they found that a woman who smokes a pack a day or more has a 42 percent higher risk than a nonsmoker.

What about men? A subsequent study found that male pack-a-day-or-more smokers had a 94 percent higher risk of type 2 diabetes—nearly double that of a nonsmoker.

Now, if you're thinking that smokers may have a lot of other bad habits that may lead to diabetes, the Harvard group thought the same thing. But the numbers I've just reported are true even after accounting for numerous other health risks.

A more recent analysis looked at the results of many different studies of smoking and diabetes and found a connection in 24 out of 25. Conclusion: People who currently smoke more than 20 cigarettes a day have, on average, a 61 percent higher risk of developing diabetes; former smokers, 23 percent higher.

You might think it odd that smoking can lead to diabetes. I did, too. The link seems to be that smoking causes systemic inflammation, and that same inflammation is considered a contributor to diabetes. Former smokers have less inflammation, so if you're not a "never," be a "former."

Soda: Make This Switch to Quench Diabetes Risk

Over the past few years, there's been a lot of suggestion in books and magazines that diet soda is just as bad for you as regular soda—maybe worse! One study done at four different major health centers came up with the conclusion that drinking diet soda on a daily basis was associated with a huge 67 percent greater risk of developing diabetes.

In contrast, another study that looked at consumption of regular sugar-sweetened soda found that people who gulped the most—about one or two servings a day—had a 26 percent higher risk of diabetes than those who rarely drank soda.

Which makes diet soda worse than regular soda—if you believe the statistics. Which I never did.

And later research proved my hunch was right. Diet soda was pronounced "innocent" of promoting diabetes. But regular soda was convicted of what I'd call a "nutritional felony."

Researchers at Harvard Medical School set out to examine the association between drinking sugar-sweetened beverages—soda included—and risk of type 2 diabetes in women. Their study included over 90,000 women and tracked them for 4 years.

The findings? Compared with women who drank less than one sugary soda or fruit juice per month, those who drank one or more a day had an 83 percent greater chance of developing type 2 diabetes. Further, over that 4-year period, weight gain was highest among women who increased their soda consumption from one or fewer drinks a week to one or more a day.

The researchers even factored in increases in other kinds of foods and snacks (including red meat, french fries, and sweets), levels of exercise, smoking, and other lifestyle issues. But it all came down to sweetened drinks, the study said.

We've been working up to a finding like this for over half a century. Back in 1942, the American Medical Association warned against consuming too much added sugar. At that time, soft drink bottlers were turning out 90 servings (8 ounces each) per person—less than two per week. By 2000, they were producing 600 servings per person—nearly two a day!

Back Away from the Can . . . and Reverse Your Risk

If you're at risk of diabetes, even if you don't know it, every bottle of soda you drink could be pushing you closer to the diagnosis you don't want.

I was shocked—depressed, even—to learn from a very recent study that nearly half of people with diabetes—45 percent—still drink regular sweetened soda. But even scarier was the finding that among those who didn't know they had diabetes until a test revealed it, 60 percent drank soda!

The average soda drinker with diabetes is consuming about 1½ drinks a day and taking in an average of 202 extra calories a day—just from the sugar in soda! The undiagnosed folks were guzzling even more sugar.

Think what 200 unneeded, nonnourishing calories do to your weight. Every 10 additional calories you consume (and don't burn off with more exercise) eventually turn into 1 more pound. So we're looking at carrying 20 extra diabetes-encouraging pounds, just from drinking soft drinks.

Is swilling all that soda—which today represents the single largest source of calories in our diet—a major risk factor for both obesity and diabetes? Decide for yourself, and then examine your own drinking habits.

If you're on the borderline—perhaps you've been told your blood sugar is a tad high or that you have prediabetes—stop the soda habit this very minute and you could reverse the danger you face! With all the options to soda, including water, plain seltzer, flavored seltzer, and unsweetened tea, as well as diet drinks, quitting soda seems like one of the easiest steps you can take to control your weight and defend against diabetes.

TV: Drop Your Diabetes Risk in an Hour!

Maybe *As the World Turns* should have been called *As the World Just Sits There*. A fascinating recent study looked into the relation between TV watching and weight gain. Scared *already*?

Among thousands of women followed for 6 years, each additional 2 hours of TV viewed correlated with a 23 percent higher risk of becoming obese . . . and a 14 percent higher risk of developing diabetes.

And it wasn't just that they were sitting instead of jogging. That same amount of time spent sitting at work instead of TV watching was linked with only a 5 percent higher risk of obesity and a 7 percent higher risk of diabetes.

Evidently there's something about TV watching that's especially harmful—simultaneous snacking, perhaps, or not burning calories while banging away on a keyboard. The researchers went on to do some intriguing calculations. Had the women spent those same 2 hours of extra TV time standing or walking around, they would have dropped their risk of obesity by 9 percent and their risk of diabetes by 12 percent.

The researchers said that if the women had added 1 hour of brisk walking a day, their risk would have gone down a lot more—24 percent lower for obesity and 34 percent lower for diabetes. They concluded by estimating that 30 percent of new cases of obesity and a stunning 43 percent of new cases of diabetes could be prevented by a more active lifestyle. Their definition of an "active lifestyle"? Less than 10 hours a week of TV and 30 minutes a day of brisk walking.

It's logical to suspect that maybe it's not the TV watching that encourages diabetes. Maybe TV addicts are more overweight, less active all day long, older, or smokers—all risk factors for diabetes. Only that's not true. A study in which nearly 38,000 men were followed for 10 years found that even when all those factors were taken into consideration, men who watched the most TV were still more than twice as likely to develop diabetes as men who watched least. How much TV were the high-risk men watching? More than 40 hours a week, which works out to a little more than 5½ hours a day.

You'll never hear that on your favorite TV news show. But more than doubling your risk of diabetes by watching lots of TV is not a trivial danger. If you're a big-time TV fan, you need to get a hobby that doesn't involve a remote control.

Vinegar: A Daily Drizzle Tames Blood Sugar

You may want to have some vinegar every day even if you're not concerned about your sugar levels. But before I tell you why, let's look at how vinegar can help keep your after-meal blood sugar spikes— known as postprandial hyperglycemia—under control.

Research into vinegar has been going on for years, much of it by

Carol Johnston, PhD, RD, a professor of nutrition at Arizona State University. She found that giving about 2 teaspoons of vinegar to people with insulin resistance, a danger sign of future diabetes, lowered their blood sugar response to a bagel meal by a huge 64 percent. It also increased their after-meal insulin sensitivity by 34 percent—an excellent sign. In people with type 2 diabetes, the reduction was just a 17 percent drop—some help but not much. (Dr. Johnston also found that vinegar pills or pickles didn't help.)

Later research at the Diabetes Center of Athens University Medical School came up with a more positive role for vinegar—but only when taken before certain kinds of meals. The researchers had people with type 2 diabetes consume vinegar before two different meals. One was low glycemic (meaning it tends to drive blood sugar slowly and not very high) and featured whole grain bread and lettuce. The vinegar did nothing to reduce sugar levels.

But when the people consumed vinegar and then ate a high-glycemic meal featuring mashed potatoes, there was a terrific difference. The vinegar "appetizer" reduced the total rise of blood sugar from 311 units to 181—a drop of 42 percent—compared with having the meal without vinegar.

The moral seems to be that if you're going to eat foods that drive up blood sugar quickly—like potatoes, white bread (especially a baguette, the French specialty that has the highest glycemic index of all breads), or a sweet dessert—a vinegar kickoff could help control the short-term effects on your blood sugar.

What about a person with type 1 diabetes who's taking insulin to "cover" his carbohydrates? Researchers worked with a group of people with type 1 and fed them a breakfast consisting of bread, butter, cheese, turkey ham, orange juice, and a cereal bar (75 grams of carbohydrate) and had them inject an appropriate amount of fast-acting insulin beforehand. Even with the insulin, those who had a vinegar drink before the meal had a 20 percent lower rise in blood sugar. The researchers were impressed enough to suggest that 2 tablespoons of vinegar before a meal might be a good idea even for people taking insulin.

No one wants to drink plain vinegar—it could actually choke you—so the way to go is to have a salad with vinaigrette dressing that contains about 2 tablespoons of vinegar. Since a daily salad with olive oil is a centerpiece of the Diabetes Rescue Diet, you won't have to do anything terribly unusual.

And, as I hinted before, there's another reason for doing this. A really good one.

Researchers at Harvard studied a large group of women over several years and found that, compared with women who rarely ate salads, those who enjoyed a salad with an oil-and-vinegar dressing nearly every day had less than half the chance of being stricken with fatal heart disease!

Vision: Pop This Herb to Protect It

Anyone with diabetes is advised to get regular eye exams, and a major reason for this is the danger of diabetic retinopathy. This problem is characterized by leakage from capillaries in the retina of the eye and the buildup of plaque. It can lead to blindness. Tight control of your blood sugar can help protect your eyes, but there's evidence that an herb may be of major help.

Pycnogenol is a standardized extract from a French maritime pine and is known to strengthen capillaries. In one study, patients with retinopathy were given either doses of the herb (50 milligrams three times a day) for 3 months or a placebo (inactive pill). In those who did not get the herbal treatment, retinopathy "progressively worsened during the trial and visual acuity decreased," according to the researchers.

The Pycnogenol group "showed no deterioration of retinal function and significant recovery of visual acuity." That's just one trial. But a study published in *International Ophthalmology* looked at a total of five clinical trials and reported that "all unequivocally showed that Pycnogenol retains progression of retinopathy and partly recovers visual acuity."

You might want to talk to your eye specialist about this. If he or she is not familiar with this treatment, one of several possible references would be a study in the *Journal of Ocular Pharmacology and Therapeutics*, "Pycnogenol Improves Microcirculation, Retinal

Edema, and Visual Acuity in Early Diabetic Retinopathy," which your physician can find online.

Vitamin D: The One You Need Most

The Diabetes Rescue Diet, with its large amounts of vegetables, fruits, legumes, beans, and other healthy foods, is loaded with vitamins and minerals. But there's one vitamin you may need more of. In fact, I would say it's the single most important vitamin for anyone concerned about diabetes.

Good evidence shows this nutrient may help prevent the earliest stages of blood sugar problems; help block diabetes itself; and, if you have diabetes, improve your blood sugar control. And chances are, you aren't getting enough of it to reap all these benefits.

That vitamin is vitamin D. Maybe it should be called vitamin Diabetes!

And it seems to do its good work at even the earliest stages of trouble—often called prediabetes, in which blood sugar is somewhat high but not high enough for a diagnosis of diabetes. In a study of some 12,000 people tested in the National Health and Nutrition Examination Survey, those adults in the bottom one-fourth of vitamin serum levels had a 47 percent higher risk of having prediabetes than those in the top fourth.

Just to be sure it was the relative lack of vitamin D that made this great difference, the researchers ruled out the effects of 16 other factors that might distort results—such as age, weight, or smoking—before arriving at this finding. It certainly seemed that vitamin D itself, and nothing else, was protecting those who had the higher levels.

How important is that? Considering that nearly one in four adults in the United States has prediabetes, I'd say we're looking at something with huge potential to curb the diabetes epidemic gripping the nation!

Diabetes Risk Cut in Half!

Doctors from major health centers in Boston tested more than 600 women who were newly diagnosed with diabetes and compared them with an equal number of women—matched for age—who did not have diabetes.

Finding: Women who tested in the top fourth for vitamin D levels were only half as likely to have diabetes as those in the bottom fourth. It's a long journey from Boston to the remote Faroe Islands, which lie off the northwestern coast of Scotland, but much the same thing was found there. Examining an older group of Faroese, as they're called, doctors found that those with low levels of vitamin D had double the risk of being newly diagnosed with diabetes.

"Double the risk" in folks with low vitamin D is the flip side of the "half risk" for people with high vitamin D, as found in Boston. Do you agree we're on to something here?

In Australia, they found the same thing: The more vitamin D, the less the risk of diabetes. Case closed!

Low Vitamin D Drives Up Blood Sugar and Complications

What about people who already have diabetes? Are they low in vitamin D? And is that harming them? It certainly looks that way!

One medical clinic examined 459 diabetes patients and found that 60.8 percent had seriously low levels of vitamin D, compared with 40.8 percent of patients without diabetes. More to the point, diabetes patients with low vitamin D had higher levels of A1c glucose, the

---

A Common D-ficiency

Based on a study of a very large number of Americans, researchers estimated that nearly three out of four adults (and adolescents) had insufficient levels of vitamin D. A recent article in *Endocrine Practice* puts the number of people with insufficient levels even higher—77 percent! Older people are at especially high risk because as we age, our skin loses the ability to use the energy of sunlight to make vitamin D.

And people who are obese (one-third of the population) have low levels of active vitamin D because it's locked inside their fat tissue.

Is Every Heart Attack Victim Low in D?

Close to it, according to a report in the *American Journal of Cardiology* that was published the same day I was writing this! A study carried out in 20 US hospitals checked vitamin D levels in 239 patients who had been admitted with acute myocardial infarction—heart attack. (Remember that people with diabetes have double or more the risk of heart disease as people without it.)

Finding: Seventy-five percent of these patients were deficient—extremely low—in vitamin D. Another 21 percent had insufficient levels. Altogether, 96 percent of these heart attack victims had "abnormally low" vitamin D levels! Furthermore, people with diabetes in this group were more likely to be in the cellar for vitamin D—absolutely deficient.

Good to know if you have your vitamin levels checked: The sufficient amount mentioned in the above study is 30 nanograms or more per milliliter.

long-term measurement of blood sugar levels. The higher your A1c, the greater the risk of complications.

And those with low vitamin D did in fact have complications—a higher prevalence of cardiovascular disease, body inflammation, and a tendency for dangerous blood clotting. The authors note that these findings fit in well with other studies showing that low vitamin D is associated with higher prevalence of arterial calcification and heart attack. I found it interesting that women were more likely to have low D than men, according to the doctors.

That study was published in 2006. In 2010, a study of thousands of Americans found essentially the same thing: The lower the vitamin status, the higher the levels of A1c blood sugar—even in people who did not have diabetes.

Putting Vitamin D to the Test

If you're wondering why everyone isn't being told to have their levels of vitamin D tested or to simply take supplements as a safety measure, it's because one thing is lacking from the whole picture. And that's a large, long-term "intervention" study in which people are told to take vitamin D, followed for years, and then tested for prediabetes, diabetes, A1c, and other factors.

In April 2011, a small, short-term, promising-looking intervention study appeared in the *American Journal of Clinical Nutrition*. Noting the evidence that links vitamin D to glucose metabolism, the researchers arranged to have 90 people with diabetes consume extra vitamin D for 12 weeks—long enough for any difference to show up on an A1c test of blood sugar.

Some of the participants consumed a twice-daily yogurt drink fortified with 500 IU of vitamin D, for a total of 1,000 IU per day. Others had plain yogurt, while still others had a drink with the same amount of vitamin D but also extra calcium.

The winner was yogurt with extra vitamin D, with or without the extra calcium. People who drank it, compared with those who had plain yogurt, had significantly improved A1c levels, lower fasting glucose, and improved insulin resistance.

Since I have yogurt nearly every morning and take my vitamin D at the same time, I feel pretty good about this finding. We'll have to wait to see what effect it has on "official" recommendations for diabetes management.

Obviously, it's hard to get enough vitamin D from either food or sunlight—otherwise so many wouldn't be lacking (see "A Common D-ficiency" on page 325). Government guidelines suggest getting 400 to 600 IU of vitamin D a day, with the amount going up with age. But there is a growing consensus that these amounts are too low.

In a study that tracked some 83,000 nurses for 20 years, researchers found that vitamin D from food had no protective effect on diabetes, but vitamin D from supplements did. They also found that calcium, from both food and supplements, had a protective effect.

They went on to nail down the exact amounts of both that are associated with protection against diabetes. Women who had a daily intake of more than 800 IU of vitamin D and more than 1,200 milligrams of calcium from food and supplements had a 33 percent lower risk of diabetes than other women who got lower amounts—400 IU of vitamin D and less than 600 milligrams of calcium. Note that less than 800 IU of D did nothing to help matters. That's crucial, because the official recommendations for vitamin D are 400 IU a day for adults and children age 4 and older.

One expert recently suggested 1,000 IU or more as a reasonable intake. That happens to be exactly how much I take every morning. Why? Because that's what my endocrinologist told me to take. Blood tests revealed that, like many people, I was on the low side of D, and he didn't like that.

Talk to your own doctor and see what he or she thinks you should do about vitamin D. The possible benefits from being well stocked on D are too important to ignore.

Vitamin Pills: Which Ones May Be Useless—Or Even Harmful

Vitamins are great—vitamins from food, at least. But when it comes to taking extra vitamins in pill form to stave off diabetes or its complications, supplements pretty much bombed out in several large studies.

One study looked at more than 125,000 female and male health professionals and their dietary habits for 12 years. No meaningful link was found between taking multivitamin pills and the subsequent risk of developing diabetes.

Perhaps you're thinking, "Well, all those doctors and nurses were probably eating a good diet, and maybe they didn't need extra vitamins." That's what I thought.

A larger study, which involved nearly a quarter of a million average older folks, looked at the use of multivitamins, individual vitamins, and incidence of diabetes over a 5-year period. These researchers, too, found no relation at all between the multis and risk of diabetes. Among individual vitamins, there were also no differences, except for a small reduction of risk from vitamin C and calcium. (Vitamin D, perhaps significantly, wasn't looked at.) That's not to say taking vitamins wasn't doing these folks good—but it wasn't doing much to block diabetes.

What if you assigned one group of people to take vitamins, instead of just observing what they were doing by inclination? Researchers tried that with more than 8,000 female health professionals, all over the age of 40. Half took vitamin C, vitamin E, and beta-carotene (a precursor to vitamin A), and the others took inert look-alike pills. Nine years later, there was zero statistically significant difference between the two groups regarding type 2 diabetes incidence.

Moral (to me, anyway): Vitamin pills don't do much to prevent diabetes. It's food that does all the heavy lifting, as in the Diabetes Rescue Diet. The one exception might be vitamin D, but even that isn't certain.

In the food versus vitamin pill showdown, it's worth mentioning that in the study above of health professionals, generous consumption of the mineral magnesium was related to a substantial reduction in risk of diabetes—but only in food form. Supplements of magnesium offered no real protection. But you'll get plenty of protection with the Diabetes Rescue Diet's whole grains, nuts, and green leafy vegetables.

Taking Vitamin C? Be Careful!

People with diabetes tend to have lower levels of vitamin C than other people. And a study we mentioned earlier (see "Vitamin C: Fruity-licious Diabetes Protection" on page 101) found that people with high levels of vitamin C in their blood have a seriously lower risk of developing diabetes.

If that gives you the idea of taking high levels of vitamin C in supplement form to bolster your protection, hold on a minute. It could be downright dangerous.

In the Iowa Women's Health Study, nearly 2,000 postmenopausal women, all of whom were diabetic, were tracked for 15 years, with their diets and health monitored. At the beginning of the study, all women were free of coronary heart disease (CHD). By the time the study ended, there was a surprise finding: Women who had the highest intakes of vitamin C from food and supplements experienced twice the occurrence of CHD and stroke as those with the lowest intakes.

Now, before you decide to toss out your oranges, here's the key point: Analysis showed that the risk came only from vitamin C in supplement form, not food. Even high consumption of C from foods had no ill effect. It was the supplements that seemed to cause the higher risk. And only at certain doses—specifically, amounts of 300 milligrams a day or more. Another important point: No such relationship was found among women who did not have diabetes when the study began. Apparently, people with diabetes have to be more cautious when choosing supplements.

To be sure these results weren't blaming vitamin C unjustly, the researchers adjusted the numbers to account for a host of other factors, such as age, weight, duration of diabetes, even the kind of medication the women were taking. Still, there was a risk of heart disease about two times higher in the high-dose vitamin C takers versus those who took none.

Selenium—Also Under Suspicion

Selenium is a trace element that, like vitamin C, acts as an antioxidant, so it's also used as a supplement. A 2007 report in the *Annals of Internal Medicine* suggests that taking it might not be a great idea if you want to avoid diabetes.

A study divided 1,200 people into two groups. One was assigned to take 200 micrograms of selenium a day, while the other group took a placebo—an inert pill. Seven years later, those taking the selenium were 55 percent more likely to have developed diabetes than those who didn't take it. Making the connection stronger, those with the highest levels of selenium in their blood plasma were between 2½ and 3 times more likely to have developed diabetes.

The Recommended Dietary Allowance for selenium is 55 micrograms a day, and you should get all you need from the Diabetes Rescue Diet's grains, fish, poultry, and nuts. Brazil nuts have a weirdly high level of selenium, so you should eat them less frequently than other nuts.

If you're wondering about the effect of relatively low doses of C, the study showed that women who took less than 100 milligrams a day actually had a slightly lower heart disease risk than those who took none.

The authors of this study take note of the fact that vitamin C is an antioxidant, which is supposed to counteract biochemical processes—oxidative stress—that hurt the body and are more common in people with diabetes. So what went wrong? They speculate that while vitamin C in foods is "balanced biochemically" by other factors in the food, a vitamin in chemical form is not balanced and may act differently, at least in people with diabetes.

Me, I don't take any supplemental vitamin C at all, because I believe the Diabetes Rescue Diet gives me what I need. If I did take C, I'd keep the daily amount under 100 milligrams, based on this study. The US Recommended Dietary Allowance for vitamin C is 75 milligrams a day for women and 90 for men. With all the natural food, fruits, and vegetables in the Diabetes Rescue Diet, you should meet and exceed that amount easily.

If you're unsure about taking vitamin C, talk to your doctor or a registered dietitian.

Water: Sip to Slash Hospital Stays

If you're in the senior citizen age bracket, you probably know that it's important to avoid dehydration, because—among other reasons—as we grow older, our sense of thirst becomes weaker. But maybe you didn't know that if you have diabetes, you have a higher-than-average risk of "running on dry"—and maybe sputtering to a halt!

Dehydration is a real threat for any senior. One study found that nearly 7 percent of all Medicare hospital admissions listed dehydration as one of the causes. Back in 1991, Medicare reimbursed $446 million for hospital admissions where dehydration was the primary diagnosis. That was a long time ago; we could easily be talking billions of Medicare dollars spent on treating dehydration today. So it's your patriotic duty to keep your water tank filled!

Often, dehydration occurs when other health problems, such as an infection, are present. But it can catch up with even the hale and hearty. This was driven home to me some years ago when my healthy, trim, active father-in-law collapsed from dehydration on the golf course on a hot day. Hours in the hot sun can suck you dry.

A person with diabetes is at higher risk, and if your blood sugars are running high, the risk is greater, because that makes you lose water. During a 1995 heat wave in Chicago, people with diabetes had a 30 percent "excess" admission to hospitals.

And the sun isn't the only danger. During the winter, cold, dry air entering your home pulls water out of your skin. Some drugs, like certain blood pressure medications, also tend to dehydrate you.

You may have heard the "rule" that you should drink no less than 8 glasses of water a day. There's no real science backing that up, though. The Mayo Clinic suggests that a glass with every meal and one between meals will probably be enough under normal circumstances. Golf, tennis, hikes, and long outings on a fishing boat or picnic are another matter and call for extra fluids—before, during, and after. The idea is to sip-sip-sip rather than chugging down one big drink and thinking you're okay.

Even with that, it's best to avoid long periods outdoors when the temperature climbs into the 80s.

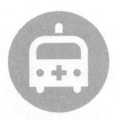

12 Healthy Bonuses

Beyond Diabetes Prevention
and Management

Most diets are aimed at one or two purposes—among them: weight loss, heart protection, blood pressure reduction, and diabetes prevention and control. And while there's a different diet for each condition, most of us are trying to prevent or deal with more than one, if not all, of these health troubles.

The diet described in this book is unique in that it achieves all those key health goals—and more! As you browse the following pages, I think you'll be amazed to see how many "bonus" benefits you stand to gain from the traditional Mediterranean diet, on which our Diabetes Rescue Diet is based. Some benefits, like lower blood pressure, may not surprise you. But how about upping your protection against cancer? Relieving inflammation? Enjoying better sex? I believe this is the first time all these research-based facts have been brought together in one place. Taken as a whole, it suggests there is something about our diet that promotes total health—from the brain to the feet— more than any other. I'm sure you will agree!

Big Healthy Bonus No. 1:
Increased Cancer Protection!

You know that diabetes raises your risk of heart disease, high blood pressure, vision problems, and more, but few people realize that diabetes also raises the risk of cancer. A person with diabetes has up to twice the risk of six kinds of cancer than the average person. The reason for this is not known.

Can the Diabetes Rescue Diet—derived from the traditional Mediterranean diet—help protect you from this danger? The answer is *absolutely*! And not by a little but a *lot*.

A 2004 research article in *Public Health Nutrition* reported that people who eat the most vegetables and fruits have a 30 to 70 percent reduced risk of cancers of the digestive tract. That high rate of protection against cancers of the stomach, colon, and more was found in the folks who were in the top third of produce consumption. You know by now that eating more produce is at the very core of the Diabetes Rescue Diet, so you'll be entering the safer zone with no extra effort—a free but very valuable bonus!

I never heard of the term *aerodigestive tract* until I read a report that looked at the effect, if any, of the Mediterranean diet on the parts of the body that are involved in both breathing and digestion. The researchers devised a simple questionnaire that gave points for following the eight most basic parts of the Mediterranean diet. The people who had at least six "yes" answers on the quiz were found to have 60 percent less cancer of the mouth and pharynx, 74 percent less cancer of the esophagus, and 77 percent fewer cases of cancer of the larynx. How's that for a bonus?

Cancer of the lungs is one of the most common cancers, and we've all been told that the one thing to do is to stop smoking or even move out of the house if anyone in there smokes. What I think you have not heard is that following our diet plan also has a very powerful protective effect. In a study that looked at the relationship between lung cancer and components of the diet, researchers found that eating relatively generous amounts of foods key to the Diabetes Rescue Diet clearly provided protection.

★ Sage used regularly—57 percent lower risk

★ Tomatoes—41 percent lower risk

★ White meat (poultry)—34 percent lower risk

★ Carrots—33 percent lower risk

★ Olive oil used exclusively—33 percent lower risk

All these foods are exactly what you'll be eating more of as you follow the Diabetes Rescue Diet. As for the sage, sprinkle it in cooked beans, fish, chicken, and pizza.

Breast Cancer Protection? Yes!

What about breast cancer, specifically? The answer is yes, there is a lot of protection in your new diet. Doctors in Spain compared 100 women with breast cancer who were admitted to a hospital to 100 women admitted for other problems to see if there was a diet connection.

It turned out to be—no surprise—fruits and vegetables. Women who ate the least veggies had nearly four times the risk of cancer as those who ate the most. The doctors also found that women with the highest levels of vitamin C (a sign of eating lots of produce) had a 60 percent lower risk, while those who had the highest intakes of monounsaturated fats (probably from olive oil, since this was in Spain) had a huge 70 percent lower risk.

A US study carried out in western New York State found similar results. Premenopausal women, age 40 years or older, who ate the most vegetables had a 54 percent lower risk of breast cancer. Interesting add-on fact: Taking supplements that contain certain nutrients found in produce, like vitamin C and folic acid, were not connected with protection from breast cancer.

Once again, you'll see that the key foods apparently involved in breast cancer protection are the very same ones emphasized in the Diabetes Rescue Diet. So as you defend yourself against diabetes and its complications, you enjoy as a bonus this great extra protection.

The Harvard School of Public Health and the Athens University Medical School carried out another investigation of the link between breast cancer and diet. Their results were almost identical to the other studies. They concluded that "vegetables and fruits are inversely, significantly, and strongly associated" with the risk of breast cancer. For you non–English majors, *inversely* means going in opposite directions. The more fruits and vegetables, the less breast cancer.

They also found that olive oil was protective. More than one serving a day cut risk by 25 percent!

Skin Cancer Risk Reduced

Skin cancer is the most common malignancy in the United States, and the deadliest type is cutaneous melanoma. It's the sixth leading cause of cancer deaths and increasingly common.

Again, it looks like the Mediterranean diet—parts of it, anyway—could offer protection. In a study that compared the dietary habits of women admitted to a hospital with or without cutaneous melanoma, doctors found that women who regularly ate fish, especially fatty fish, plus lots of fruits and vegetables were about half as likely to develop the cancer as women who ate the least.

To make sure the results weren't distorted by differences in sun exposure, that was factored in, along with skin pigmentation. So even when complexion and sun exposure were the same, diet difference offered apparent protection.

Is All This Protection Just a Coincidence?

I had to wonder—maybe you do, too: Is it some kind of strange coincidence that the very same foods that defend against diabetes and its most common complications, like heart disease, also protect against cancer?

But I've concluded that it's no coincidence at all. As you've read in this book, this same diet defends us from a whole host of diseases and ailments—everything from obesity and high blood pressure to Alzheimer's disease and, yes, even death.

I believe there is something about this pattern of eating that promotes total health in ways we don't yet fully understand. But at least we understand how to reap its benefits!

Big Healthy Bonus No. 2: Better Sex!

Do you have type 2 diabetes? Would you like to enjoy sex more—or more often? Then the Diabetes Rescue Diet is for you, according to a pair of recent studies that focused on the sexual complications of diabetes. (Not surprisingly, both studies were conducted by researchers from Italy, known for its people's enthusiasm for *amore*.)

Men and women with type 2 diabetes tend to experience sexual problems. For example, men are more likely to have erectile dysfunction (ED), defined as a consistent inability to have an erection firm enough for intercourse. In fact, men with diabetes are two to three times more likely to have ED than men who don't.

Women with type 2 diabetes tend to develop sexual issues as well. One study found that 42 percent of diabetic women experienced problems like decreased vaginal lubrication, pain or discomfort during intercourse, or no sexual desire or arousal.

Regardless of gender, these sexual complications occur because of the damage diabetes can wreak on blood vessels and nerves, including reduced bloodflow.

But you can enjoy more satisfying sex simply by following the delicious, hearty, Mediterranean way of eating. That's the conclusion of the studies mentioned above, which included more than 1,000 men and women with type 2 diabetes. These studies, both led by researchers at the Second University of Naples, investigated how following a

Mediterranean-style diet (rich in whole grains, fresh fruits and vegetables, dried beans and other legumes, olive oil, and nuts and fish, with a reduced intake of red or processed meat) impacted rates of ED (in men) and sexual function (in women). Let's look at each study separately.

The first study looked at more than 550 males with diabetes ranging in age from 35 to 70. The researchers used a 9-point scale to assess how closely the men's diets followed the Mediterranean ideal. The higher the score, the better.

The men with the highest scores (6 to 9) generally had less body fat, smaller waists, and fewer problems with obesity and metabolic syndrome. They also tended to be more physically active and have healthier cholesterol and blood sugar levels. Further, only 52 percent of the men following the Mediterranean diet suffered from ED, compared with 62 percent of those who did not.

In the case of severe ED, only 16.5 percent of those following the Mediterranean diet suffered from it, compared with 26.4 percent of those who did not. The Mediterranean-style eaters were also more likely to be sexually active.

The second study assessed sexual function in almost 600 women with diabetes. They also ranged in age from 35 to 70, and the researchers used the same 9-point scale to assess their diets. Again, higher scores showed that they followed the Mediterranean diet more often.

The results virtually mirrored those of the men's study. Women with the highest scores—again, 6 to 9—carried less body fat, had smaller waistlines, and were less likely to be obese or have metabolic syndrome. They also tended to be less depressed and more physically active and have healthier levels of cholesterol and blood sugar.

Further, women who "ate Mediterranean" most often had the lowest prevalence of what researchers call sexual dysfunction—issues centered around sexual desire, arousal, lubrication, orgasm, satisfaction, and pain.

So along with preventing or managing diabetes, reducing your risk of cardiovascular disease, and losing belly fat, you'll enjoy more and better lovemaking. That's no surprise. After all, the Mediterranean way of life is all about pleasure—and lovemaking ranks right up there on the pleasure scale, whether you're from Italy or Indiana!

Big Healthy Bonus No. 3: Lower Blood Pressure!

High blood pressure is both a major risk factor for and common complication of diabetes. As many as two out of three people with diabetes have high blood pressure, according to the American Diabetes Association. And a study in the *British Medical Journal* found the risk of diabetes complications was "strongly associated with raised blood pressure." Clearly, defending yourself is important, whether you're trying to avoid the condition or currently have it. Following the Diabetes Rescue Diet will be a major help in that regard.

As reported in the *Journal of Hypertension,* a study of 2,000 men and women older than 18 found that "consumption of a Mediterranean diet was associated with a 26 percent lower risk of being hypertensive." Among those with high blood pressure, there was "a 36 percent greater probability of having blood pressure controlled."

An article published in the *Journal of Clinical Hypertension* notes that the Mediterranean diet has been found to reduce the risk of heart disease (as we spelled out in Part 1) and poses the question: Could lower blood pressure be involved in the protection?

One study, the author reports, found that the diet's defense against atherosclerosis—clogged arteries—was "mainly due to lower levels of blood pressure and body mass index [degree of fatness]." Another study that compared people who had had a first heart attack with a similar group that had not found that the higher the score on the Mediterranean diet, "the lower the risk of a heart attack, mainly due to lower blood pressure levels."

So it seems clear that the Med-style diet tends to prevent high blood pressure and overweight, both risk factors for heart disease.

Two of the "pillars" of the Diabetes Rescue Diet are greater consumption of fruits and vegetables. Are they important for protection? A large study published in the *British Journal of Nutrition* examined

4,400 people to see how many had undiagnosed high blood pressure and then checked their habitual diets. Finding: Those who were in the highest quintile (20 percent) for eating fruit had a 32 percent lower risk of being hypertensive—and not knowing it. The highest vegetable eaters had a 42 percent lower risk. Best of all, those who ate plentiful amounts of both fruits and vegetables had a tremendous 77 percent lower risk of undiagnosed high blood pressure.

You should be able to move to the head of the fruit-and-vegetable class effortlessly on the Diabetes Rescue Diet. Considering how common high blood pressure is and the difficulties people experience controlling it, we have here another big bonus!

P.S. Get your blood pressure checked regularly.

Big Healthy Bonus No. 4:
Easier (and Tastier) Weight Control!

The Diabetes Rescue Diet does not emphasize weight loss as a primary way to improve your overall protection. As I pointed out at some length earlier, weight-loss programs have a pathetically low rate of success, with even poorer results among people with diabetes. Yet it's helpful not to put on excess pounds as the years roll by. The great thing about this diet is that it seems to prevent obesity automatically—a wonderful "side effect," you might say.

In a study of more than 3,000 people, age 18 all the way to 89 years old, people who most closely followed the Mediterranean diet were found to be less than half as likely to be obese as those whose diets were not Mediterranean. And there's no need for perfection to get this protection: Just being in the top one-third is enough to do the trick.

The Med-type eaters got a bonus, too. Besides being 51 percent less likely to become obese, they were 59 percent less likely to have "central" obesity—lots of belly fat, which is especially bad if you're trying to avoid diabetes.

Weight Gain Stopped in Its Tracks!

A study of more than 10,000 university graduates in Spain found that those whose diets were closest to the Mediterranean style gained the least weight over a 4-year period. And compared with those whose diets were the least Mediterranean, they were 24 percent less likely to have gained more than 10 pounds.

Another study confirms that a Mediterranean-style diet can help stop obesity in its tracks. Following tens of thousands of men and women for 3 years, researchers found that overweight people who most closely followed a Mediterranean diet were up to 30 percent less likely to become obese than people with other diet styles.

Weight Loss Our Way

Tested head-to-head against the commonly prescribed low-fat diet, we made the opposition look kind of pathetic. In an 18-month weight-loss program involving 100 overweight men and women, half were randomly assigned to a low-fat diet and half to a moderate-fat Mediterranean-style diet. The actual percentages of fat were 20 in the low-fat group and 35 in the Mediterranean. All the participants ate reduced-calorie diets.

After 18 months, the Mediterranean-style dieters, on average, lost 9 pounds and took $2\frac{3}{4}$ inches off their waists. The low-fat dieters, ironically, got fatter! They gained more than 6 pounds and added about half an inch to their waists.

One of the reasons for this shocking disparity is that by the end of the program, only 20 percent of the low-fat group were still actively participating, while 54 percent of the Mediterranean group were still going strong.

Was it superior tastiness that made that big difference? That's my guess. But the numbers speak for themselves: a total 15-pound advantage to the weight-loss winner—Mediterranean style!

Healthier Weight Loss for Diabetes!

Another head-to-head test of the usually recommended low-fat diet versus a Mediterranean diet for weight loss was carried out at Ben-Gurion University of the Negev in Israel. This was a very structured test that lasted all of 2 years—much longer than most diet trials. At its conclusion, the low-fat dieters had lost an average of $6\frac{1}{2}$ pounds, while those who ate Mediterranean style lost an average of 10 pounds. Good! But wait, there's more.

Among the dieters who had diabetes, those following a low-fat diet actually increased their fasting blood sugar levels an average of 12 milligrams, while those following the Mediterranean diet lowered theirs by 33 milligrams.

More weight lost and a major difference in blood sugars—45 "points"! You don't have to be an endocrinologist to appreciate what that means to a person with diabetes.

Big Healthy Bonus No. 5:
Better Spirits and a Healthier Brain!

Keeping the dangers of diabetes at bay and protecting your heart are important, but then there's the question of mental and emotional well-being. Can the diet I'm recommending help you in those departments, too?

The answer is especially important to people with diabetes, who have a higher-than-average risk of mental problems. Fortunately, the answer is yes, it can help, according to research—and to an astonishing degree.

One study concluded that people whose diets most closely matched the traditional Mediterranean diet—on which the Diabetes Rescue Diet is based—had a much lower risk of developing depression than those eating different diets. The risk reduction was as high as 51 percent.

Would you ever imagine that simply using more olive oil—as you do on this plan—could help make you a happier person? Me neither. But apparently, it can.

A study followed nearly 5,000 people for 10 years, looking at their diets and testing for presence or absence of severe depressed mood (SDM, it's called). It's not a rare condition: Over the course of the study, 11 percent of men and 16 percent of women developed it. The researchers discovered that women who consumed the most oleic acid (the fatty acid found richly in olive oil) were less than half as likely to develop SDM as those who consumed the least. Not too bad—for a salad dressing!

A Younger, Sharper Mind!

Even the happiest of us begin to worry about declining mental sharpness when we qualify for senior citizen discounts. But you can worry less if you're eating your salads, olive oil, fruits, and the rest.

The Chicago Healthy Aging Project measured cognitive decline (loss of mental sharpness) in a large group of folks over the age of 65 and then looked at their diets. What they did was score each person's usual food intake to see how closely it matched up with either the Mediterranean diet or something called the Healthy Eating Index (a scoring system used by the US government to measure adherence to their Dietary Guidelines for Americans).

Finding: Seniors who followed our diet the closest had less than average mental decline, while those who ate more in tune with the Dietary Guidelines showed no such advantage. Lead study author Christine Tangney, associate professor of nutrition at Rush Medical College in Chicago, said those in the top third of adherence to the Mediterranean diet had the mental sharpness of someone 2 years younger.

Rescue from Alzheimer's

What would you do to lessen your risk of developing Alzheimer's disease? Would you follow the dietary program in this book? Because that could help a lot!

Researchers at New York's Taub Institute for Research on Alzheimer's Disease and the Aging Brain worked with doctors from the Departments of Neurology and Medicine at Columbia University. They looked for any possible relationship between following the Mediterranean diet and the occurrence of Alzheimer's disease (AD). They divided seniors into three groups, ranked for diet patterns that had low, medium, or high resemblance to the Mediterranean style. Compared with those with a low match, those in the medium group had a 53 percent lower risk of AD and those in the top third, 68 percent—more than two-thirds—lower risk.

Importantly, the researchers also investigated to see if this apparent protection was perhaps due to the presence or absence of other

Foods That *Clobber* Your Brain
If You Have Diabetes!

An international study published in 2009 examined the effect of fat consumption on the rate of cognitive decline among nurses with type 2 diabetes, age 70 and over. The bombshell discovery was that generous consumption of a certain kind of fat is like whopping your head with a ball-peen hammer (not exactly the words of the researchers)!

The damage is caused by trans fatty acids. While small amounts are found in natural foods, three-quarters of our intake comes from hydrogenated and partially hydrogenated vegetable oils, especially in snack and junk foods.

Women who were in the top one-third for trans fat consumption did much worse on six different tests of thinking ability, compared with those in the bottom third. How much faster were they "losing it"? The difference was "comparable with the difference we find in women 7 years apart in age," according to the researchers.

Imagine losing 7 years of mental youth because of poor food choices! Or, to look at it in a more positive way, imagine escaping the loss of 7 years of mental aging by eating right!

Trans fats are added to foods mostly to increase shelf life and stabilize flavors. Check food labels and simply refuse to buy anything containing trans fats. The main sources are commercially manufactured cakes, cookies, crackers, pies, potato chips, and corn chips—all excluded from the Diabetes Rescue Diet.

health problems, such as diabetes, heart disease, stroke, or high blood pressure. It wasn't. It was the diet.

In 2007, the same group did further research, which was published in the medical journal *Neurology*. This time they looked at people who had developed AD to see how high they scored for following a Mediterranean diet and how long they lived. Those in the medium group had a 35 percent lower risk of dying during a follow-up of 4.4 years, compared with the lowest scoring. Those with the highest scores had a dramatic 73 percent lower risk! The authors noted that the Mediterranean diet may affect not only the risk of AD but the "subsequent disease course" as well.

A further study looked at how likely seniors with mild cognitive impairment were to develop AD. The researchers discovered that those in the top third of Mediterranean-style eating had a 38 percent lower risk than those in the bottom third. They also noted that the this protective dietary pattern featured a high intake of salad dressing, nuts, fish, tomatoes, poultry, crucifereous vegetables (like broccoli and cauliflower), fruits and dark green leafy vegetables and a low intake of high-fat dairy, red meat, organ meat, and butter. If you've read the first part of this book, you'll realize this is the exact diet pattern of the Diabetes Rescue Diet.

Stroke Danger Greatly Reduced

One possible reason for the Mediterranean diet's apparent power to protect against Alzheimer's disease is that it might prevent cerebrovascular infarcts—strokes that kill part of the brain through blockage of bloodflow and oxygen and may contribute to AD.

In a 2011 New York study published in the *Annals of Neurology*, hundreds of people over the age of 65 who'd been scored for how closely their diets resembled the Mediterranean style were given magnetic resonance imaging (MRI) scans years later, and the incidence of infarcts was recorded. Seniors whose diets were moderately adherent were 22 percent less likely to have had an infarct than those in the lowest third. Those in the top third of adherence to the diet were 36 percent less likely to have had an infarct.

You already know that a stroke can disable or kill a person, so this bonus of AD protection is clearly major!

Your Brain Enjoys a Nice Walk

Regular walking is a key component of the Diabetes Rescue Diet. It's great for defending against diabetes and a host of other problems, but it will also help keep your brain in tip-top shape.

I recommend several hours of walking a week. That should make a big difference. According to one study, older women who walk as little as 1½ hours a week at an easy pace have "significantly better cognitive function and less cognitive decline" than women who walk less than 40 minutes weekly. Not too bad for just 90 minutes of walking a week!

Big Healthy Bonus No. 6:
More Magnesium,
the Antidiabetes Mineral!

What with all the fruits, vegetables, whole grains, beans, and low-fat dairy in the Diabetes Rescue Diet, you know you'll be getting a heaping helping of vitamins and minerals. But one mineral deserves special mention.

It's so obscure and underrated that it isn't even listed on nutrition labels. Most people (except readers of *Prevention* magazine) have probably never heard of it. It's called magnesium, and scientists are almost calling it the anti-diabetes mineral. One study conducted at the Chapel Hill campus of the University of North Carolina found that people who eat the most magnesium have just half the risk of developing diabetes as those with low levels.

In another study of nearly 36,000 "older" Iowa women, researchers looked for dietary factors that affected the chance of developing diabetes over a 6-year period. No surprise at two of the findings: Eating lots of whole grains was linked to a 21 percent lower risk and lots of fiber to a 22 percent lower risk. But women who got the most magnesium in their diets had a 33 percent lower risk of being diagnosed with diabetes.

In an even larger study involving more than 100,000 men and women tracked for 12 to 18 years, men who got the most magnesium had a 33 percent lower risk of developing diabetes, and women, 34 percent—exactly the same protection seen in two different studies!

Still another study looked at magnesium in younger folks—18 to 20 years old—and compared it with the appearance of the metabolic syndrome, a cluster of problems including impaired blood sugar control and considered a major warning sign of impending diabetes and/or heart disease. The high-magnesium people had a 31 percent lower risk than the low-magnesium group. So all three studies show almost the same effect: about a full one-third lower risk with plentiful magnesium.

Magnesium at Work for You in the Diabetes Rescue Diet

I'm pointing out all these studies in Big Healthy Bonuses because you'll automatically get lots of magnesium by following this plan. As one of the study authors points out, whole grains, nuts, and green leafy vegetables are excellent sources of magnesium. And they're all featured front and center in our diet.

The safest-from-diabetes intake of magnesium for a person on an average 2,000-calorie-a-day diet is about 400 milligrams. To get an idea of exactly where you'll find the most magnesium in your new diet and, for comparison, some poor sources, check out the table below.

FOOD	MAGNESIUM (IN MG)
Brazil nuts 1 oz (6–8)	107
Quinoa, ½ cup, cooked	89
Raisin bran, 1 cup	83
Spinach, ½ cup, cooked	79
Halibut, 3 oz	78
Black beans, ½ cup, cooked	61
Peanut butter, 2 Tbsp	50
Flat fish, 3 oz	49
Navy beans, ½ cup, cooked	48
Brown rice, ½ cup, cooked	42
Cucumber, 1 large	34
Shrimp, 3 oz	29
Whole wheat bread, 1 slice	24
Pumpernickel bread, 1 slice	17
Rye bread, 1 slice	13
White rice, ½ cup, cooked	13
Corn Chex, 1 cup	8
White bread, 1 slice	6

Do you see the tremendous difference between whole grain breads and white? White, of course, is not part of the Diabetes Rescue Diet. With so much important nutrition removed in the refining process, it doesn't belong in any health-promoting diet. The same goes for rice. And breakfast cereals!

Big Healthy Bonus No. 7:
Increased Protection
against Limb Loss!

Following the Diabetes Rescue Diet can greatly reduce your risk of one of the most feared complications of diabetes—the need to have a leg amputated.

At a hospital center where such procedures were done, doctors noted that 48 percent of patients had diabetes. Their risk of amputation was 10 times higher than that of people without diabetes.

Importantly, the researchers recorded that more than 94 percent of people needing amputation had severe peripheral arterial disease, or PAD. PAD is obviously bad news. It involves blockage of the arteries supplying the legs and, according to one expert, "is associated with a marked increase in the short-term risk of heart attack, stroke, amputation, and death." And it affects more than 8 million Americans.

Following the diet this book is all about can go a long way toward avoiding PAD. A study in Italy found that when comparing diabetes patients with or without arterial complications, those who most closely followed a Mediterranean diet were 56 percent less likely to have PAD—less than half the risk.

Big Healthy Bonus No. 8:
Breathe Better, Breathe Longer!

Ever hear of chronic obstructive pulmonary disease, also known as COPD? Chronic bronchitis and emphysema are two common forms of this disease, for which there is no cure. Shockingly, considering it's a problem you don't hear much about, COPD is actually the fourth leading cause of death in the United States. Johnny Carson died of COPD.

Remarkably, the Mediterranean diet pattern reduces the risk of COPD by half. In a study of 43,000 men followed for 12 years, those who ate the most fruits, vegetables, whole grains, and fish were 50 percent less likely to be afflicted by COPD than men who ate a Western diet, which has lots of processed foods, refined sugars, and red and processed meats. Men whose diets were least Mediterranean were 4 times more likely to develop COPD over the 12 years. Why all this food-related protection against a disease caused in large part by smoking? Doctors speculate that a Mediterranean-style diet is especially rich in those factors, such as vitamins and antioxidants, that ward off all manner of disease, from cancer to diabetes to lung disease.

Big Healthy Bonus No. 9:
Prevent or Relieve
Rheumatoid Arthritis!

Rheumatoid arthritis (RA) is a condition in which the body's own immune system attacks itself—especially the joints. Most of its victims are women, at least in the United States. There are treatments to relieve the pain and stiffness, but no cure.

The good news: promising evidence that key elements of the Diabetes Rescue Diet may work to prevent RA or relieve the symptoms in people who have it.

Researchers from Harvard Medical School and the University of Athens Medical School looked at the health and diet histories of hundreds of people in southern Greece to see if there was any connection between 100 different foods, how frequently they were eaten, and the incidence of RA. They found just two strong associations: People who consumed generous amounts of either olive oil or cooked vegetables had less risk of RA. Both foods are, of course, central to the diet this book is devoted to.

People who were in the highest category of consuming cooked vegetables were 76 percent less likely to have RA than those who ate the least. For olive oil, there was a 62 percent lower risk.

But what if you purposely gave people who already had RA a more

Mediterranean diet? Would it help? Investigators in Sweden had a group of patients with RA (all well controlled with drugs) eat either a Mediterranean-style diet or a typical Western diet for 12 weeks. It took 6 weeks for improvements to set in, but by the end of the trial, patients on the Mediterranean diet had "a reduction in inflammatory activity, an increase in physical function, and improved vitality," according to the researchers. Those on the ordinary diet saw no improvements.

A more recent study that involved a larger number of people, all women, found the same results in participants who were given Mediterranean meals and hands-on classes on how to prepare fresher, healthier foods.

Why the protection? Researchers don't know exactly but suggest that the natural anti-inflammatory power of olive oil, as well as the antioxidants in the entire diet pattern, may be involved.

Big Healthy Bonus No. 10:
A Lower Risk of Gallstone Disease!

Surgery to remove gallstones is common. It's estimated that more than 20 million Americans have gallbladder disease, with women developing it twice as often men. Can the Diabetes Rescue Diet afford you any protection? It can, if you remember to include the nuts we talked about earlier!

A study of 80,000 women who were followed for 20 years found that women who ate an ounce of nuts (or peanut butter) at least 5 times a week (just as we suggest) had a 25 percent lower risk of requiring surgery for gallstones, compared with those who rarely ate nuts.

A different study followed a large group of men and looked at the relationship between nut consumption and the diagnosis of gallstone disease. Men who ate their 5 ounces of nuts a week had a 30 percent lower risk than men who rarely ate nuts—another nice bonus of the Diabetes Rescue Diet!

The olive oil component of our diet may also help. A report published by the Rhode Island Medical Society points out that olive oil "enhances gallbladder emptying, reducing cholelithiasis [gallstone] risk."

Big Healthy Bonus No. 11: Asthma Relief for Kids and Grown-Ups!

Asthma is increasing worldwide, and no one is sure why. Could diet be involved?

Researchers from Spain and the National Institute of Public Health in Mexico investigated the presence of asthma symptoms in Mexican children, ages 6 to 7, and their nutrition habits over a 1-year period.

When scores were given according to how closely the diets of kids with and without asthma matched up with a Mediterranean-style diet, a strong protective effect was discovered. Children who had the closest match were 40 percent less likely to have asthma; 36 percent less likely to wheeze; 37 percent less likely to have itchy, watery eyes; and a very impressive 59 percent lower risk of having rhinitis (sneezing and runny nose). The authors suggest that eating less junk food helped, too.

Studies of children in Spain and Crete found similar results—less wheezing with a diet rich in vegetables, fruits, fish, and other parts of our diet. Noting these results, a research team from Portugal and Finland set out to see if adults might also benefit from the right diet. They examined 174 asthmatics and used standard tests to determine if they were controlled or uncontrolled. Then they analyzed their diets.

Remarkably, adults with asthma who had the most Mediterranean-style diets were 78 percent less likely to be uncontrolled. One of the most powerful protectors in the diet turned out to be fruit: Eating an average of 10 ounces a day of fresh fruit was linked to a 71 percent lower risk of out-of-control asthma. You can get that much fruit by eating two whole oranges, apples, pears, or tomatoes or half a pint of strawberries a day.

Big Healthy Bonus No. 12: Stronger, Thicker Bones!

First thing to know: All older women are at risk of bone fractures, but women with type 2 diabetes have nearly twice the risk of women without diabetes. Women with the more unusual type 1 diabetes have a fracture risk seven times higher.

I doubt you knew that, because it's rarely talked about.

I'm going to talk about it because the Diabetes Rescue Diet will help you avoid the pain, disability, and medical costs of broken bones. Hip fractures are considered the "most devastating" of all fractures. And they aren't rare—more than 350,000 occur each year in the United States, and that number is rising rapidly.

Here's how you'll Rescue yourself: Just follow the walking part of our plan!

A study of more than 61,000 women, 40 to 77 years old, found that those who walked (and got no other exercise) reduced their risk of suffering a hip fracture by a very impressive 41 percent. They achieved that protection by walking just 4 hours a week or more—right in line with the Diabetes Rescue's recommendations for preventing and controlling diabetes.

The Swedish Hip Fracture Study Group also found that a little physical activity goes a long way toward keeping bones in one piece. Looking at how much recent time was spent in leisure physical activity, they discovered that a little is good, and more—terrific.

Women who exercised a little, but not more than 1 hour a week, had 21 percent less risk of winding up with a broken hip, compared with the totally sedentary. Women who were active 1 to 2 hours a week had a 33 percent lower risk. And women who managed to be active for 3-plus hours a week cut their risk by more than half.

Imagine—just a few hours a week of walking or gardening can cut your risk of a broken hip in half! You'll get that much activity easily on this plan.

Are you a senior? In a study of 9,700 women at four different health centers in different states, researchers found that "moderately to vigorously active women" 65 and older had a 42 percent lower risk of hip fracture.

All this is an added bonus benefit you get with the Diabetes Rescue Diet. Entirely aside from diabetes, I think you'll agree that it's worth every step you take!

Index

||||||||||||||||||||||||||||||||||||||||

Underscored page references indicate boxed text and tables.

B

Bacon, health risks from, <u>135</u>
Baked goods, olive oil in, 48
Bananas
    Breakfast Biscuits with Fruit
        Spread, 167
    Strawberry-Banana Crepes, 241
Barley
    Minestrone Soup with Barley, 192
    uses for, 37
    Wild Rice and Barley Pilaf, 223
Basil
    Shrimp with Garlic, Basil, and
        Fennel, 212
Beans
    alternatives to, <u>92</u>
    Butter Beans in Fresh Tomato
        Sauce, 220
    canned, <u>90</u>, 93, 143
    Crispy Tuscan-Roasted Chickpeas, 236
    in dip, 47–48
    dried, preparing, <u>90</u>, 93, 94
    gas from, preventing, 93–94
    health benefits of, 23, 85–93
    Hummus, 94, 231
    Lamb Stew with Chickpeas and
        Bulgur, 217
    Pasta Salad with Tuna, Eggs, and
        Red Beans, 182
    Poblano Chile and Bean Soup, 193
    recommended intake of, 85, 93
    Refried Beans, 221
    Tabbouleh with Chickpeas and
        Artichoke Hearts, 179
    Turkey–Black Bean Burgers, 188
    types of, <u>88–89</u>
    uses for, 85, 94–96, 143
    Warm Taco Bean Salad, 175
    whole vs. refried, <u>95</u>
Beef
    ground, 138–39
    lean, choosing, 137, <u>138</u>
    Orange-Beef Stir-Fry, 216
    Veggie-Stuffed Meat Loaf, 214–15
Beets
    Roasted Beet, Apple, and Walnut
        Salad, 181
Belly fat
    foods reducing
        beans, <u>86</u>
        olive oil, 39, 41
        peanuts, 63, 66
        whole grains, 31, 33

    health risks from, 39, 41, 253–54
    Mediterranean diet preventing, 340
    walking for losing, 253–55
Berries. *See also specific berries*
    Fresh Berry-Oat Muffins, 168
    health benefits of, 103–6
    Panna Cotta with Berries, 247
Beverages. *See also specific beverages*
    sweetened, consumptionn of, 120
Biscuits
    Breakfast Biscuits with Fruit
        Spread, 167
Blackberries, 106
Blindness, from diabetes, 3
Blood fats. *See also* Cholesterol levels;
    Triglycerides
    Mediterranean diet improving, 14
    reviewing, before walking program,
        259
    whole grains lowering, 23, 25
Blood pressure. *See also* High blood
    pressure
    in metabolic syndrome, 9
    reducing, with
        berries, 103
        Mediterranean diet, 10
        nuts, 62
        omega-3 fats, 23, 50
        walking, 255
Blood sugar control
    in diabetes
        decline in, 12
        difficulty of, 3
        vitamin D for, 324
    diabetic peripheral neuropathy and,
        315
    for eye protection, 323
    foods for
        beans, 23, 86–87, 88, 91, <u>95</u>
        mushrooms, 73, 74, 76
        nuts, 62–63, <u>64</u>
        red wine, 112–14
        sourdough, rye, and pumpernickel
          bread, <u>30</u>
        vinegar, 321–23
        whole grains, 23, 25
    from loss of belly fat, 254–55
    Mediterranean diet for, 10, 14
Blood sugar levels
    checking, before and after walks,
        259
    checking, with alcohol consumption,
        119
    controlling (*see* Blood sugar control)